The SLP's IDEA Companion™

by Shaila Lucas

Content Area	Ages	Grades
■ student management	■ 5 through 17	■ K through 12

Evidence-Based Practice

■ According to the Individuals with Disabilities Education Act (IDEA) (2004), an individualized education program (IEP) should include:

- a statement of the child's present levels of academic achievement and functional performance, including a description of benchmarks or short-term objectives of children with disabilities who take alternate assessments

- a statement of measurable annual goals, including academic and functional goals

- a description of how the child's progress toward meeting the annual goals will be measured

■ The American Speech-Language-Hearing Association (ASHA) recommends that speech-language pathologists (SLPs) continue to identify short-term goals as part of their intervention plans in order to monitor progress toward long-term goals. As we strive toward improved evidence-based practice in our profession, it is clear that we should maintain documentation of treatment effectiveness (ASHA, 2006).

The SLP's IDEA Companion incorporates these principles and is also based on expert professional practice.

References

American Speech-Language-Hearing Association (ASHA). (2006). *IDEA Part B final regulations: A side-by-side comparison analysis.* Retrieved July 21, 2009, from asha.org/advocacy/federal/idea/idearegactivity.htm

Individuals with Disabilities Education Act (IDEA). (2004). Retrieved July 21, 2009, from idea.ed.gov

LinguiSystems

LinguiSystems, Inc.
3100 4th Avenue
East Moline, IL 61244
800-776-4332

FAX 800-577-4555
Email: service@linguisystems.com
Web: linguisystems.com

Printed in the U.S.A.

ISBN 10: 0-7606-0321-9
ISBN 13: 978-0-7606-0321-5

About the Author

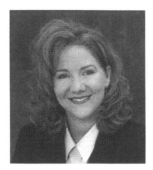

Shaila Lucas, M.S., CCC-SLP, is currently a speech-language pathologist with the Saugus Union School District. She has a special interest in promoting the efficacy of speech pathology through outcome measures. Shaila presents frequently on topics pertinent to speech pathology and education. She is a graduate of California State University, Northridge, where she received a master's degree in 1996. She resides in Saugus, California, with her husband Lonnie and puppies Mario and Biscotti. *The SLP's IDEA Companion* is her first publication with LinguiSystems.

Acknowledgments

I wish to extend my appreciation to the following professionals whose expertise shaped the methodologies presented in this book:

June Haerle Campbell, M.A., CCC-SLP — Northwestern University
Eileen James, M.A., CCC-SLP — Kaiser Permanente
Charlene Boshart, M.A., CCC-SLP — Speech Dynamics
Elizabeth Weber, Ph.D., CCC-SLP — California State University, Northridge

Edited by Barb Truman
Illustrated by Margaret Warner
Page Layout by Christine Buysse
Cover Design by Lyle Hart

Table of Contents

The SLP's IDEA Companion is a valuable tool as you write instructional goals according to the new IDEA guidelines. Use the benchmarks provided in *The SLP's IDEA Companion* as a guide for writing benchmarks specific to your individual students. If your needs require benchmarks to be worded in true behavioral format, you may need to add the following information:

1. when the benchmark will be reached
2. how progress will be measured
3. what media will be used to meet the benchmark
4. who will complete the benchmark
5. what task will be completed
6. what criteria or proficiency will be reached
7. who will help the student achieve the benchmark

For example, the benchmark "The student identifies the main idea of a paragraph" could be written as follows:

By May 30, 2004, when presented with a written paragraph from his social studies text, the student will identify the main idea of the paragraph with 90% accuracy in ten trials. The student's mother, his classroom teacher, and his speech-language pathologist will help him achieve this benchmark.

Table of Contents, *continued*

Introduction

The Individuals with Disabilities Education Act (IDEA) has recently undergone several changes that directly affect the procedures of the practice of speech pathology in the school setting. It is important to be aware of these changes because they impact how goals are written and measured, how the level of a student's performance is determined, how progress is reported, and how assessments are conducted. *The SLP's IDEA Companion* helps the school-based speech-language pathologist (SLP) meet several of the directives set forth in IDEA '97. The following is an explanation of the changes and how *The SLP's IDEA Companion* can assist you in meeting the required components of the new law.

Goals and Benchmarks

General Education currently uses benchmarks to implement local and state standards. Benchmarks are statements about reference points along the path toward learning a new skill or set of skills. They are identified sub-skills that are required to meet the desired standard. IDEA '97 requires that Special Education use benchmarks too. Each IEP must now include a measurable goal(s) and the benchmark(s) or short-term objective(s) used to measure progress toward meeting the goal(s). The benchmarks can be taken directly from the content area (i.e., curriculum) or modified to target functional skills which are prerequisite to meeting the expectations of the curriculum. For example, a sixth grade language arts content standard may state, "… the student expands listening vocabulary." This is a very appropriate goal for a student with a language impairment. Often the basic skills required to meet this goal, however, (e.g., inferring the meaning of an unknown word) are not spelled out. In this case, benchmarks are written to indicate any intermediate steps needed to help a student with a language impairment reach the overall goal (e.g., expanding listening vocabulary). To create meaningful goals and benchmarks, you need to be familiar with the areas of the core curriculum that are based on a proficiency of language and, therefore, troublesome for a student with language deficits.

The SLP's IDEA Companion provides goals and benchmarks taken from the curricular areas most likely to be in deficit for a student with a language impairment. These goals and objectives come from several states' content standard areas (i.e., core curriculum) and specifically target listening, speaking, language arts, study skills, math, and literature. *The SLP's IDEA Companion* is a "short-cut" to these areas. It provides classroom expectations from kindergarten through 12th grade, organized in nine distinct areas of communication:

- Fluency
- Narrative/Expository
- Oral-Motor/Articulation
- Phonological Awareness
- Pragmatics
- Semantics
- Syntax
- Voice
- Word-Finding

The benchmarks in each of these areas are worded so that they can be adapted to fit district and/or individual student needs. Specific criteria which may be added include:

- under what circumstances the behavior will occur (e.g., after a prompt, independently, in the classroom setting)
- the criteria of measurement (e.g., 4/5 times, when directed by the clinician)
- the time parameter in which the benchmark will be reached (e.g., by the first quarter; by March, 2000)

Since specific content standard areas for speech (e.g., fluency, voice, articulation) do not exist, the overall goals for these areas are classroom based, but not necessarily the benchmarks needed to reach the goal. It is advisable, however, to use classroom material as the basis for intervention, stating so on the IEP (e.g., using core curricular material the client will state the main idea 4/5 times).

In deciding which benchmarks are appropriate for a student, realize that the classroom teacher's input can help you prioritize the most important language skills to address. It is often the case that targeting a specific area (e.g., listening comprehension) that the teacher has identified as most problematic is more effective than working on skills based on standardized testing alone.

Level of Performance

The new IDEA adds another requirement to the IEP, stating that there be a "Present Level of Educational Functioning." This statement should reflect at what level the student is successful (e.g., "Sarah is currently using syntactical structures at the second grade level."). This level should clearly indicate a starting point for intervention. If the student has been receiving services, the statement should reflect the growth the student has made in the target area until that point in time. The Present Level of Functioning also should include how the student's disability affects his/her classroom performance (e.g., "Sarah's delay in syntax affects her ability to understand passive relationships, use complex sentence structures, and understand the purpose of sentences."). These statements serve to coordinate the goals of the classroom teacher and the specialist. If the student is of preschool age, the statement outlines how the disability affects participation in appropriate activities such as using speech to communicate basic needs or using rising inflection to request information.

Although the classroom teacher can give you much valuable information about a student's area of deficit, it is often more difficult for the teacher to provide a more specific level of functioning. This is especially true in the area of oral expression. Standardized tests can give some indication of a level, but they are usually not grade specific. Since *The SLP's IDEA Companion* provides baseline measures for each goal, these baselines can be used to establish at what level the student's language "breaks down." Once an area of focus is determined (e.g., syntax), you can administer several baselines of a benchmark at a level where you think the student is generally functioning. For example, if the student is in third grade and is having significant trouble with the oral and written structure of language, collaborate with the classroom teacher to find out which benchmarks might be appropriate for the student's needs. Then administer several baselines of those benchmarks to gauge the level of functioning. The level at which the student has difficulty with the baselines is a good starting place for intervention. If the baselines are too simple, advance the level to find the "breaking" point where the skill is weak (e.g., the student is successful one out of three times).

When writing goals for a student in the upper grades, guidelines, rather than specific baselines, are provided to help you judge if a benchmark has been met. For example, in the area of narrative skills, instead of providing 10 baselines of high-school level length narratives, a checklist-type format is provided to help you determine if the benchmark is appropriate. This should be more useful in the interest of time.

Report of Progress

The revised IDEA states that the IEP must include a statement of how progress toward annual goals will be measured (e.g., criterion-referenced tests, standardized tests, teacher-made evaluation, teacher observation, or other measures specified on the IEP). This addition to IDEA is important because it requires a "system" be in place for measurement purposes.

The Act further mandates a report of how parents will be regularly informed of progress, most likely in the form of periodic report cards. Special Education is now required to report progress at least as often as Regular Education.

It may be difficult at times to determine whether or not a student has met a particular benchmark. Usually you are working in small groups, using cues and scaffolding to assist the student in building a new skill. This environment, while appropriate for learning, doesn't always lend itself to pinpointing an amount of growth. To facilitate this task, the baselines included in *The SLP's IDEA Companion* are sample questions of each benchmark measure. Baselines used to determine a starting point for therapy can be re-administered to assess growth. Alternately, the baselines can be used to affirm clinical judgment of the progress the student has made. As a "teacher-made evaluation" tool, the number of "trials" to administer is left to your clinical judgment.

Assessment

In the area of assessment, IDEA '97 states that triennial standardized testing is no longer required (although many individual school districts have their own guidelines). At the time of the reevaluation, it should be determined by the IEP team if the need for more data exists in order to establish eligibility criteria. If the team concludes that the student continues to meet eligibility criteria, no further assessment is needed. In this case, other forms of appropriate evaluation tools can be used to assess progress just as for annual IEPs.

Since reevaluations do not require standardized testing, baseline measures can be used in the same manner as when determining the next step of intervention for a student. This may be an increase in the grade level of a skill in an identified area or a decrease in the support needed to achieve a particular benchmark. This change in testing due to IDEA '97 should reduce paperwork and the time dedicated to testing.

It is my hope that *The SLP's IDEA Companion* meets your needs as you strive to blend the "clinic" and the "classroom" — providing a clear correlation between communicative disorders (especially language impairments) and reading and writing deficits. Because school-based SLPs understand the demands of communication in the classroom, we have the unique opportunity to affect a student's academic success, and furthermore, his or her self-worth. May you find joy and fulfillment as you better the lives of students for whom communication is a challenge.

Shaila

8

Fluency

Although fluency skills are not directly addressed in the core curricular standards, disfluent speech can have a significant impact on a student's academic progress. Stuttering detracts from a student's verbal message, drawing adverse attention to his speech. Furthermore, the emotional repercussions of stuttering can hinder involvement in class discussion, cause uncertainty in oral presentations, and possibly lead to social withdrawal from peers.

The benchmarks and baselines in this unit provide intervention strategies ranging from less to more specific. The less specific approaches in the Borderline/Mild Disfluency section (pages 10 – 17) focus on home environment changes, fluency shaping techniques, and resisting time pressure. Use your clinical judgment to decide whether or not to include the parent program in your benchmarks. Although the less specific approach is written for borderline to mild stuttering behaviors, you might find it helpful for students who stutter severely as well. Use the more specific strategies in the Moderate to Severe Disfluency section (pages 18 – 23) if the less specific strategies are insufficient in helping a student manage fluency or if an emotional component needs to be addressed.

Fluency

Borderline/Mild Disfluency

Parent Program

> **Goal:** to modify environmental factors contributing to disfluency through parent education and training

Benchmark 1: The parent differentiates between typical disfluencies and stuttering behavior when demonstrated by the clinician.

Baseline 1: Ask the parent to identify the following disfluencies as typical disfluencies or stuttering behavior.

Statement	*Classification*
"Get the bay baby."	stuttering behavior (syllable repetition)
"I want mmmmany."	stuttering behavior (prolongation)
"Please please let me go."	typical disfluency (whole word repetition)
"I um, um will."	typical disfluency (interjection)
"Does she-he like to sing?"	typical disfluency (revision)
"I w-(tense pause)-ant some."	stuttering behavior (block)
"S-s-s-soon it will rain."	stuttering behavior (sound repetition)
"Where (pause) are you?"	typical disfluency (hesitation)

Benchmark 2: The parent identifies factors which tend to disrupt fluency by charting disfluent episodes and reporting to the clinician.

Baseline 2: Say to the parent:

"Tell me how you would find out if a specific factor was a 'fluency disrupter' (i.e., making your child stutter)."
> *Target:* Observe that behavior over time and chart the child's speech (e.g., during "spotlight" talking or while the child is upset).

"What kind of factors have you found to be fluency disrupters?"
> *Target:* hurried schedule, competition to talk, illness, anxiety, etc.

Benchmark 3: The parent develops a problem-solving approach to minimizing fluency-disrupting influences at home, in school, and in social settings, and reports to the clinician.

Baseline 3: Say to the parent, "What changes at home, in school, or in social environments help to minimize fluency-disrupting influences?"
Target: used more pause time, spent "quiet time" with my child, gave teacher information, etc.

Benchmark 4: The parent spends undivided listening time with his child on a daily basis as reported to the clinician.

Baseline 4: Say to the parent, "How many times a week are you able to spend at least 10 minutes of quiet, listening time with your child?"
Target: daily

Benchmark 5: The parent develops communicative models conducive to fluency development (e.g., more relaxed speech, more pause time, quiet listening) and describes them to the clinician.

Baseline 5: Say to the parent, "Demonstrate or describe what you do to help your child talk easier."
Target: slow speech, pausing, listening without interrupting, etc.

Benchmark 6: The parent supports his child's generalization of said strategy through completion of home practice programs as reported to the clinician.

Baseline 6: Say to the parent, "Describe activities you do with your child to help him practice "easy talking" (or target strategies such as "smooth movements" or "turtle talking").
Target: card games, describing pictures, or any other activities suggested by the clinician

Student Intervention Program

> **Goal:** to increase fluency through speech modification techniques

Benchmark 1: The student uses a fluency-shaping technique to repeat words, phrases, and sentences modeled by the clinician.

Baseline 1: These types of fluency goals are best measured as a student completes a particular skill level in therapy. It may be best to administer a baseline after each level is achieved instead of at each reporting period. Some common fluency-shaping terms and techniques are:

easy talking   stretching
easy beginnings   soft contacts
easy onset   turtle talking
smooth movements

Say to the student, "Repeat after me using _____ (easy beginnings, easy onsets, etc.)."

Words

mug	digging
bike	teacher
sunset	desk
crab	judge
apple	cheese

Phrases	*Sentences*
red cars	Red cars are easy to see.
a bird	A bird sits on a fence.
purple monsters	Purple monsters eat cherry pie.
many colors	Many colors are used in painting.
the swings	The swings squeak when they move.
fast runners	Fast runners win races.
bright stars	Bright stars can be seen on a clear night.
heavy rocks	Heavy rocks are hard to lift.
a part	A part of the cake has been eaten.
sunny days	Sunny days are my favorite.

Benchmark 2: The student uses a fluency-shaping technique to name pictures.

    Baseline 2: Provide the student with noun pictures and say, "Name these pictures using (technique)."

Benchmark 3: The student uses a fluency-shaping technique to produce a word in a carrier sentence.

    Baseline 3: Provide the student with noun pictures and say, "Use (technique) as you say, 'I see a _____' for each picture."

Benchmark 4: The student uses a fluency-shaping technique to create a sentence about a picture.

    Baseline 4: Provide action pictures and say to the student, "Use (technique) to tell me what is happening in this picture."

Benchmark 5: The student uses a fluency-shaping technique to create complex sentences about pictures.

    Baseline 5: Provide two action pictures or one with several activities pictured, and have the student create a complex sentence about them. Tell the student, "Use (technique) to tell me what is happening in this/these picture(s)." For example, if one action picture shows a girl raking leaves and another shows a boy pulling a wagon, the target response might be, "The girl is raking the leaves, and the boy is pulling a wagon."

Benchmark 6: The student uses a fluency-shaping technique in structured conversation using student- or clinician-created topics.

    Note: The measurements on Benchmarks 6-8 depend on the technique the student is using. The focus of the modification might be on the start of a sentence (which could be measured in 4/5 sentences used), on a phrase (4/5 phrases), or on a word (2/10 words). Write the benchmark accordingly.

    It is helpful to let the student know the target frequency (e.g., 4/5 sentences).

Baseline 6: Tell the student, "We're going to practice (technique) while we talk about _____."

- our favorite family activity
- what we don't like for lunch
- why it's good to go to bed on time
- what we like to do when the weather gets cold
- the best vacation we've had (or favorite place to visit)
- why it's smart to eat a balanced meal
- what we don't like about school/work
- why we think it's a good idea to brush our teeth
- why it's important to be kind to friends
- our favorite pizza toppings

Benchmark 7: The student uses a fluency-shaping technique in transfer activities (e.g., storytelling, giving descriptions, giving directions, barrier games) with cues.

> *Note:* Cues may take the form of reminding the student to use "easy beginnings," pointing to a picture of a turtle, or verbal reinforcement (e.g., "good smooth talking").

Baseline 7: Say to the student, "Tell me _____."

- how to get from the office to your classroom
- what an elephant looks like
- about the last story you read (or your favorite story)
- the difference between a refrigerator and a freezer
- how to play a game (e.g., four-square, checkers, hide-and-seek)
- how to ride a bicycle
- how to make a peanut butter and jelly sandwich
- about the difference between a plane and a helicopter
- how you make a phone call
- how you get ready for bed

Benchmark 8: The student uses a fluency-shaping technique during spontaneous speech to produce fluent speech.

Baseline 8: This benchmark is best measured by observation of spontaneous speech. Since the overall goal with fluency-shaping is to maintain fluency over long periods of time, the modification becomes a "tool" the student can use when needed to manage fluency. Judge the benchmark as met if the disfluency has been reduced to a pre-determined "normal" level (e.g., less than 10% disfluencies).

Benchmark 9: The student uses a fluency-shaping technique to maintain fluency at levels of increasing difficulty (e.g., based on location, physical activity, persons present, listener reaction).

Baseline 9: Provide additional elements of difficulty, such as moving to another location, providing background noise, adding an additional person (e.g., adult or classmate), adding physical activity, or acting like an impatient listener while following the hierarchy of Benchmarks 1-8.

Assess the student's ability using guidelines from Baselines 1-8. The following is a method for keeping track of a student's progress. For example, when in a location outside the regular therapy session, this student was able to maintain fluency 5/5 times while repeating words, naming pictures, and using a carrier phrase, and 4/5 times when creating a sentence about a picture.

Additional Factor	*Benchmark*							
	1	2	3	4	5	6	7	8
change in location	5/5	5/5	5/5	4/5				
change in physical activity								
change in person present								
change in listener reaction								

Benchmark 10: The student evaluates his own attempt at target behavior in Baseline 9, agreeing with the clinician's evaluation.

Baseline 10: As the student performs Baseline 9, have him give feedback about his performance using a + or – and compare it to your evaluation.

Benchmark 11: The student resists time pressure by pausing when role-playing situations that simulate confrontation.

Baseline 11: Create time pressure during your role play by using rushed speech, an increased voice volume, a frustrated sigh, or an accusatory tone. Have the student play the defensive role. Say to the student, "You've been practicing pausing to give you extra time when you have to answer a question or feel pressure. Now we're going to practice pausing in some situations that might make you feel anxious."

1. **Waiter/Customer:** You're at a new restaurant and not sure what you want to order. The waiter has come back twice and acts very impatient as he says, "Are you ready to order yet?"

2. **Salesperson/Customer:** There is a broken vase on the floor beside you, but it was like that when you got there. The salesperson says, "Did you drop that vase? You know if you break something, you have to buy it!"

3. **Teacher/Student:** Your teacher is looking at your math test and says, "The answers on your test are the same as the student who sits next to you. Did you copy his paper?"

4. **Door-to-Door Salesperson/Child:** The salesperson is trying to get you to buy a calendar and you don't think you should. He says, "You really need to buy this calendar. You need one for the new year. Your mom or dad will really be glad you bought it. It's only $20. Can you go get the $20?"

5. **Parent/Child:** You borrowed your dad's favorite pen to write a note and now you can't find it. Your dad says, "Where is my favorite pen? I know you used it yesterday."

6. **Grocery Clerk/Customer:** You always buy a certain type of cereal, but the space where it usually is, is empty. You ask the clerk if they have any more in the back. The clerk says, "You need to look in the middle of aisle 12 on the left-hand side. I'm sure you'll find several boxes there." You know that's where you already looked.

7. **Friend/Friend:** Your friend wants you to loan him your bike and you don't think you should. He says, "Let me borrow your bike. I wrecked mine and I really need to get to the store. Come on. Your dad won't find out. I'll be right back."

8. **Principal/Student:** The principal saw food thrown in the cafeteria. He says, "Did you throw that piece of bread? I think it came from around here!"

9. **Neighbor/Young Person:** You are riding your skateboard down the street and a neighbor yells, "There are wheel marks on my grass! Did you ride your skateboard through my yard?"

10. **Phone Solicitor/Child:** He is trying to find out if your parents are home, and you're not supposed to give that information. He asks, "Is your mother or father home? It's really important that I speak with your mom or dad."

Benchmark 12: The student learns general relaxation exercises and explains their importance in easier talking when questioned by the clinician.

Baseline 12: Ask the student to demonstrate the exercises she's learned in therapy. Ask why relaxation is important to know how to do voluntarily.

For example:

"We've been working on ways to feel more relaxed. Tell or show me what we've practiced."
> *Target:* demonstration of exercises used in therapy; feel differences between tension in muscles and relaxed muscles

"Why is relaxation important?"
> *Target:* I can reduce the tension in my body. I tend to stutter more when I feel tense/nervous/anxious.

Moderate to Severe Disfluency

> **Goal:** to improve the ability to manage stuttering through attitude modification and speech modification

Benchmark 1: The student explains concepts related to stuttering when directed by the clinician.

Baseline 1: Ask the student to relate what he has learned about stuttering (e.g., the cause), the pattern of his stuttering, or anything that has come up in therapy.

For example:

"What is stuttering?"
> *Target:* bumps in a person's speech, getting stuck on words, interruption in my speech, when I go (stuttering behavior), etc.

"What causes stuttering?"
> *Target:* Nobody's really sure, but it has to do with a mistiming of the nerves and muscles working together to make smooth speech.

"In which situations is your stuttering better? Worse?"
> *Target:* pinpoint less/more difficult talking situations

"What kind of jobs can people who stutter do?"
> Target: anything they want

"How should/do you feel about talking?"
> *Target:* I can say what I want, when I want to.

"What happens if/when you let stuttering control what you say or when you say it?"
> *Target:* I miss out, don't get to say what I want, people don't know I'm smart, I feel bad, etc.

Benchmark 2: The student explores good and bad feelings associated with stuttering (e.g., fear, anger, embarrassment, pride) by answering questions about how stuttering affects how he feels.

Baseline 2: Talk about how the student feels about stuttering by asking questions such as:

"How do you feel when you stutter?"
> *Target:* pinpoint feelings associated with stuttering

"What happens when you feel that way?"
> *Target:* want to hide the stuttering, not talk anymore, want to try again, keep quiet in class, etc.

"What would happen if you _____ (tried to hide your stuttering, didn't talk anymore, tried again, kept quiet in class, etc.)?"
> *Target:* negative or positive consequences (being more scared of stuttering, not getting a good grade in class, etc.)

"How do you feel when you "conquer the stuttering monster," "don't let stuttering control you," "face the stuttering moment," etc.?
> *Target:* like I'm in control, proud, encouraged, feel good about myself

Benchmark 3: The student gives a class presentation about stuttering with the clinician or attends a presentation the clinician gives to his class.

> *Note:* Before you talk to the class about stuttering, make sure the student is comfortable with your doing so.

Baseline 3: Judge the benchmark as met if the activity is completed. The presentation might include how the speech mechanism works, how/why speech gets "stuck," ramifications of teasing, etc.

Benchmark 4: The student describes the anatomy involved in speech and demonstrates a knowledge about the physiology of stuttering.

Baseline 4: Ask the student what she has learned about her "speech helpers" (larynx/voice box, lips, tongue, lungs) and how they apply to fluent and disfluent speech.

For example:

"Which parts of your body help you talk/make sounds/use speech?"
> *Target:* articulators (larynx, lips, etc.)

"How does each part work?"
> *Target:* lungs provide the air, voice box provides the sound, lips and tongue shape the air

"What happens when you stutter?"
> *Target:* Something gets stuck along the way like my lip or my tongue, and the sound has trouble getting all the way out, or I stop the air when I hold my breath, etc.

Benchmark 5: The student identifies the type of stutter modeled by the clinician.

Baseline 5: Give examples of different types of stuttering. Have the student label the stutter and tell where/what stuck. The target depends on the words used to describe stuttering. For example, "Tell me what kind of stutter you hear, where the sound got 'stuck,' and which speech helper was involved."

Word	*Kind of Stutter*	*Speech Helper / Where Stuck*
l-l-l-leave	said too many times	tongue tip stuck behind teeth
mmmmoon	sound held too long	lips stuck together
k-(block)-itty	no sound	back of tongue stuck to roof of mouth
t-t-t-tie	said too many times	tongue tip stuck behind teeth
ssssandal	sound held too long	tongue stuck behind teeth
g-g-g-gate	said too many times	back of tongue stuck to roof of mouth
b-(block)-utton	no sound	lips stuck together
aaaapple	held too long	stuck in throat
sh-(block)-out	no sound	tongue stuck to roof of mouth
zzzebra	held too long	tongue stuck behind teeth

Benchmark 6: The student voluntarily produces different types of stuttering demonstrated by the clinician.

Baseline 6: Have the student voluntarily produce different types of stuttering. For example, "You stutter on some words now, and I'll guess what kind of stuttering you are using."

Target: voluntary production of sound repetition, prolongation, blocks, etc.

Benchmark 7A: The student produces words and phrases using typical stuttering behavior including any secondary characteristics she uses (e.g., facial grimaces, pitch rises, eye-blinks, tension).

Baseline 7A: Have the student purposely use the stuttering behaviors she has identified as typical for her speech as she reads or repeats words and phrases. Say, "I'm going to give/read you a word/sentence. I want you to stutter really hard on it. Use lots of tension."

Words	*Sentences*
1. tree	The tree has yellow leaves.
2. shallow	The water is shallow here.
3. missed	The arrow missed the target.
4. bank	The bank is around the corner.
5. ice cream	My favorite ice cream is strawberry.

6. walnuts   I'm allergic to walnuts.
7. fun   Playing basketball is fun.
8. checkers   My sister is good at checkers.
9. jump rope   Jumping rope takes practice.
10. restore   The dresser can't be restored.

Benchmark 7B: The student repeats the word or sentence with half the tension.

Baseline 7B: Have the student repeat the word or sentence with half the tension as used in Baseline 7A. Say, "Now ease up on the stutter. Use only half the tension this time."

Benchmark 7C: The student repeats the word or sentence with modification and explains the physical change he made to change the tension of the stutter.

Baseline 7C: Have the student repeat the word or sentence a third time using a fluency-shaping modification used in therapy. Ask the student to describe what he did physically in Baselines 7A, B, and C to change the tension.

For example:

"What changes did you make to make talking easier?"
> *Target:* I let go of some of the tension in my tongue (lips, throat, etc.) each time I said the word.

Benchmark 8: The student explains physical and cognitive analogies relating to stuttering when questioned by the clinician.

Baseline 8: Discuss the physical and cognitive analogies used to describe stuttering. Have the student explain the analogies.

For example:

"How is _____ (loosening a tight fist) like using _____ (strategy) instead of getting stuck in a stutter?"
> *Target:* You can feel the tension and then release it like easing out of a stutter.

stretching a rubber band
> *Target:* The rubber band can be changed/stretched like I can change/stretch my speech. The stretching of the rubber band is like stretching speech in an "easy beginning."

straightening a water hose with a knot in it
> *Target:* The water can move easier through the hose when there isn't a block in it.

the Chinese finger trap
> *Target:* The harder you pull, the more stuck your fingers are. It's like the harder I try to push the air out, the more stuck it gets.

blowing bubbles
> *Target:* The bubbles come out better when you blow softly and gently rather than with a fast burst of air.

Benchmark 9: The student demonstrates "cancellation" (i.e., repeating the stuttered word with modification) in stuttering moments during a structured conversation and explains its importance as a therapy tool.

Baseline 9: Talk with the student about a recent current event or school function. Instruct the student to "cancel" any hard stuttering that should occur. If no stuttering is heard, instruct the student to intentionally stutter, and then use the cancelling technique.

> *Topic Ideas*
> newspaper headlines
> new equipment on the playground
> class elections
> parent/teacher conferences
> spring/winter/summer break
> statewide testing
> recent assembly
> current art project
> cafeteria food
> traffic problems at school

Ask the student, "Why do you think it is important to 'cancel' hard stutters?"
> *Target:* I give myself another chance to use my stretching (or other strategy), and I don't have to feel bad about having a hard block or not using my fluency tools.

Benchmark 10: The student demonstrates "voluntary disfluency" (i.e., adding stuttering that occurs normally in conversational speech) during interruptions with impatient listeners and explains its importance as a fluency tool.

Baseline 10: Arrange a conversation with the student where you each have opposing viewpoints. Instruct the student to practice the tool of "voluntary disfluency."

Topic Ideas

bringing your lunch	vs.	eating at school
starting school earlier	vs.	starting school later
letting kids use a soda machine	vs.	not letting kids use a soda machine
having to wear uniforms	vs.	just having a dress code
having no homework	vs.	having homework
running a mile in PE	vs.	not running in PE
staying up until 12:00 every night	vs.	going to bed at 9:00
skateboarding on the sidewalks	vs.	skateboarding in the street
running in the hallway	vs.	walking in the hallway
having to eat all vegetables	vs.	having to eat just the vegetables you like

Ask the student, "Why is it important to 'throw in stuttering on purpose' sometimes?"

> *Target:* It puts me more in control of my speech helpers' movements when I add some stuttering on purpose. Disfluency isn't something to fear when I do it on purpose, so I feel better about my talking.

Narrative/Expository

Narrative structure draws on predictable components of story grammar. As a student gets older, his ability to recognize these elements improves as does his storytelling skills. Narratives develop from simple chains of related events to complex tales which integrate multiple plots. Character involvement moves from simple figures to intricate participants with personalities, attitudes, and agendas. In the advanced narrative, plots are no longer limited to a problem with a solution, but become mirrors of societal issues in story form.

For the students challenged with a language impairment, many elements of story grammar aren't apparent. In fact, the level of their narrative/expository skills seems to plateau at less developed stages of narrative evolution. As a result, these students don't learn to comprehend and retain spoken and written information in an efficient manner. For example, instead of fitting words they hear and read onto a framework (e.g., predictable story grammar), they rely solely on visual and auditory memory. This is an ineffective way to comprehend.

The benchmarks and baselines in this section provide transitional steps essential for students to move forward in narrative complexity. Remedial strategies such as "visualizing," which is often an underdeveloped skill for students with language impairments, are imbedded in the measures. When students are able to use imagery to mentally "picture" what they read and hear, genre such as expository language is more easily comprehended.

Many of the baselines at the grade school level are interspersed within a story. Administer those baselines which pertain to the benchmark you are interested in measuring. At the advanced grades, it is more efficient to use the student's curricular text as baseline material, measuring performance against the criteria provided. Of course grading systems will vary across districts, so feel free to modify the criteria as needed.

Narrative/Expository

Kindergarten

> **Goal:** to improve the understanding and use of the language of classroom material at the K grade level

Benchmark 1: The student places four to six story sequence pictures in chronological order.

    Baseline 1: Cut out one set of the Picture Stories on pages 125 – 134 and mix them up. Instruct the student to put the pictures in the order in which they happened.

Benchmark 2: The student uses sequence words to verbally order an event (e.g., *first, next, then, after that, last*).

    Baseline 2: Using the Picture Stories on pages 125 – 134, instruct the student to explain the order of what happened. (You may want to use the same vocabulary you used in therapy to refer to the target words. For example, "Use order words to tell the story.")

Benchmark 3: The student retells a story with visual cues (e.g., sequence cards) including problem and solution.

    Baseline 3: Using the Picture Stories on pages 125 – 134, have the student explain the story line in the picture. Judge the benchmark as met if the student includes a problem which is encountered and the solution.

Benchmark 4: The student uses descriptive language to tell stories.

    Baseline 4: Using the Picture Stories on pages 125 – 134, have the student tell a story about the pictures. (You may want to use the same vocabulary used in therapy such as "describers" or "colorful words.") Judge the benchmark as met if the student uses colors, sizes, shapes, emotions of characters, and reasons for action when describing the story.

> **Goal:** to improve the understanding and use of the language of classroom material at the 1st/2nd grade levels

Benchmark 1: The student makes an inference about a story he has read or that has been read to him.

Benchmark 2: The student identifies basic story-grammar elements (e.g., characters, setting, initiating event/problem, attempt, solution) in a story.

Benchmark 3: The student retells a story including basic elements of story grammar (e.g., characters, setting, initiating event/problem, attempt, solution) with visual or tactile cues.

> *Note:* These visual and tactile cues could be anything that gives the student a strategy for retelling the story (e.g., story map or story grammar diagram).

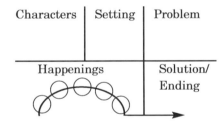

Benchmark 4: The student retells a story including basic elements of story grammar without cues.

Benchmark 5: The student creates his own story around classroom themes or curricular content.

Baselines 1-5: Read the following paragraphs to the student. Ask the question(s) (1-5) which correspond(s) to the targeted benchmark(s).

> *Note:* The baseline for Benchmark 5 (question 5) is a prompt which may not elicit a personal story from every child. Additional questioning about a child's experience may be necessary to measure this benchmark.

A. Ben's mom gave him a gift that was wrapped in colorful paper. He was very confused because it wasn't his birthday for another month. He was excited when he unwrapped it. He said, "Thanks Mom. Now I have something new to read."

1. What happened?

Ben started reading his book right away that night. He enjoyed it so much he could hardly stop reading to go to bed. The next morning he wanted to continue reading, but he couldn't find his book. He searched all over the house and finally found his sister in her room reading his book!

2. Tell me the parts of the story. (Use story mapping strategies, etc. as needed to elicit characters, setting, initiating event/problem, attempt, solution.)

3. and 4. Tell the story back to me.

5. Tell me a story about when you or someone you know was surprised. What happened?

B. Brad's stepdad saw him fall. He ran to help Brad up. "Thanks Tim," Brad said. "I won't climb that far up again."

1. What was Brad doing?

Unfortunately, Brad couldn't put pressure on his ankle when he tried to walk. His stepdad took him to the doctor who said that Brad's ankle was broken. Brad was disappointed because baseball tryouts were next week. He decided to go to the try-outs anyway. The coach said since Brad had done so well last year, he could join the team without trying out. Brad was happy.

2. Tell me the parts of the story. (Use story mapping strategies, etc. as needed to elicit characters, setting, initiating event/problem, attempt, solution.)

3. and 4. Tell the story back to me.

5. Have you ever broken a bone or known someone who has? What happened?

C. "I like my new pet," said Yoshi. It's small now, but it'll be bigger soon and it will fly all around the house."

1. What kind of pet does Yoshi have?

In a few weeks, Yoshi's bird was flying all over. One afternoon it flew into his mom's favorite plate that was hanging on the wall. The plate crashed to the floor and it shattered into pieces. Yoshi's mom was very upset and wouldn't let the bird out of the cage again.

2. Tell me the parts of the story. (Use story mapping strategies, etc. as needed to elicit characters, setting, initiating event/problem, attempt, solution.)

3. and 4. Tell the story back to me.

5. Has your pet ever gotten in trouble? What happened?

D. Ashley wanted to paint the tree house red, but Jeff wanted to paint it green. They finally painted the tree house the color Ashley wanted.

1. What color is the tree house?

Ashley and Jeff liked how their tree house looked, but one morning Ashley looked outside and saw that the rain from the night before had made the paint run off the boards and all over the grass! They had gotten the wrong kind of paint at the local hardware store. They spent the entire next day repainting their tree house with paint made for outdoors.

2. Tell me the parts of the story. (Use story mapping strategies, etc. as needed to elicit characters, setting, initiating event/problem, attempt, solution.)

3. and 4. Tell the story back to me.

5. Have you or someone you know ever had to redo something because you/they made a mistake? What happened?

E. Alex was on his way to school when he dropped a quarter in the grass. Alex looked and looked for the quarter, but he couldn't find it. At last, Alex gave up and went to school so he wouldn't be late.

1. What happened to the quarter?

Alex really needed that quarter. He wanted to buy something to drink after school, and he had just enough money before he lost the quarter. After school, he was on his way home when he found five empty soda pop cans. He turned them in at the corner convenience store and got enough money to buy his drink.

2. Tell me the parts of the story. (Use story mapping strategies, etc. as needed to elicit characters, setting, initiating event/problem, attempt, solution.)

3. and 4. Tell the story back to me.

5. Have you or someone you know ever lost something? What happened?

F. Shelly and Rosa walked out of school. They began to run, hoping to stay dry. They ran all the way home. The girls still got wet.

1. Why were the girls wet?

When they got to Shelly's house, Shelly checked in her pockets for her key. It must have fallen out while she was running. Rosa suggested they go to her house and call Shelly's mom. When they got to Rosa's house, they stood in front of the heating vent because they were really wet and cold.

2. Tell me the parts of the story. (Use story mapping strategies, etc. as needed to elicit characters, setting, initiating event/problem, attempt, solution.)

3. and 4. Tell the story back to me.

5. Have you or someone you know ever gotten locked out? What happened?

G. Anna went on a trip. Soon she was flying over the streets and trees. Everything looked so tiny. Anna looked out the window and said, "I think I can see my house!"

1. Where is Anna?

The flight attendant overheard her and asked her where she lived. When Anna gave the name of her street, the attendant said she had never heard of that street. Anna took out a map and showed her exactly where her street was. Then the attendant knew where Anna lived.

2. Tell me the parts of the story. (Use story mapping strategies, etc. as needed to elicit characters, setting, initiating event/problem, attempt, solution.)

3. and 4. Tell the story back to me.

5. Have you or someone you know ever flown on a plane? What happened?

H. Sarah saw an animal standing in a field. The animal was black and white and was chewing grass.

1. What did Sarah see?

The cow suddenly moved away from the grass it had been chewing on. Sarah realized it had seen a snake. Sarah screamed when she saw it. The snake must have been frightened by the noise because it quickly slithered away.

2. Tell me the parts of the story. (Use story mapping strategies, etc. as needed to elicit characters, setting, initiating event/problem, attempt, solution.)

3. and 4. Tell the story back to me.

5. Have you or someone you know ever been scared by an animal? What happened?

I. Rachel and Melanie had a garage sale to sell some old toys. They were hoping the money they made would be enough to replace the window. They wished they hadn't played softball so close to the house.

1. Why do the girls need money?

Rachel and Melanie bought the glass for the window and Rachel's dad replaced the broken windowpane. They had learned their lesson. They would always play softball in the park or away from houses.

2. Tell me the parts of the story. (Use story mapping strategies, etc. as needed to elicit characters, setting, initiating event/problem, attempt, solution.)

3. and 4. Tell the story back to me.

5. Have you or someone you know ever broken something valuable? What happened?

J. Mr. Jacoby was a lonely man. All the kids thought he was grouchy and mean. One day he found a stray cat wandering around in his backyard. It looked scared and hungry.

1. What do you think happened to the cat?

Mr. Jacoby brought the cat into his house. He fed it and cared for it. They became friends. The children noticed that Mr. Jacoby laughed and smiled more. They wondered why he was happy now. He said that he had a new friend.

2. Tell me the parts of the story. (Use story mapping strategies, etc. as needed to elicit characters, setting, initiating event/problem, attempt, solution.)

3. and 4. Tell the story back to me.

5. Have you ever been given something that made you happy? What happened?

> **Goal:** to improve the understanding and use of the language of classroom material at the 3rd/4th grade levels

Benchmark 1: The student creates self-monitoring questions after a set of directions have been read.

Baseline 1: Ask the student, "What are some important questions to ask yourself after you read directions?"

Target examples:
What did the directions tell me to do?
What part did I miss?
Who can I ask to find out?
Do I know what all the words mean?
Should I ask for clarification now (while teacher is speaking) or later?
Should I check to see if I got it right?

Benchmark 2: The student answers "wh" questions about story grammar elements including how the motives and emotions of characters affect the story.

Baseline 2: After the student has read (or heard) a story from curricular text, probe for comprehension about story grammar elements with the following questions:

Who are the main characters in the story?
Where does the story take place?
When does the story take place? (e.g., season, time of day, or specific year)
What is the main event in the story? Is that a problem? Why?
How is the problem solved (or attempted to be solved)?
Why do you think _____ (character) _____ (action of the character)?
How did _____ (character) feel about _____ (problem or other character)? Did that have anything to do with his/her actions?
Did _____'s (character) feelings or motives change during any part of the story? Why?

Benchmark 3: The student uses visual imagery to answer detail and inferential questions about a paragraph.

Baseline 3: As the student follows along, read the paragraphs on the next two pages. Ask questions about the details in each paragraph. Some examples are listed.

1. The two little girls sat on the cold, iron park bench as the sun set behind them. They each wore large hats, one yellow and one pink, with matching sundresses. A light breeze ruffled their skirts as they ate cotton candy.

   - What color do you picture the hats and the dresses?
   - What do you picture in the background behind the girls?
   - What do you picture the girls eating?
   - What time of day was it, morning or evening?

2. The woman's gray hair was braided. She wore glasses on her head. As she pushed her shopping cart down the bread aisle, she kept one hand on the cart. She held her list of things to buy in the other hand. One wheel of the cart was off balance, making an annoying squeaking sound.

   - What sound is in your picture?
   - What do you picture the woman doing with each of her hands?
   - What color do you picture her hair?
   - Was it easy or hard for the woman to keep her cart straight? Why?

3. The trash can lay on its side. A large brown and black raccoon picked his way through the trash, finding scraps of food in the dark. He stopped often to look around to make sure the rustling sounds of his movement didn't attract any attention.

   - How do you picture the trash can, upright or on its side?
   - What was the raccoon looking for?
   - What size do you picture the raccoon, small or large?
   - How was the raccoon feeling, confident or unsure? How do you know?

4. The storm moved over the cornfields. Sounds of thunder and flashes of lightning came from the dark clouds. Heavy rain poured down while strong winds blew the tall corn.

   - What color do you picture the clouds?
   - What movement do you picture?
   - What sounds are in the scene?
   - Where is this scene, in the city or country? How do you know?

5. The birthday cake was chocolate-covered with white icing. It had 10 candles on top. The words *Happy Birthday* were written under the candles. Around the letters were candy flowers and hearts.

   - How many candles do you picture on top of the cake?
   - What is being celebrated?
   - Do you think this cake is for a boy or girl?
   - Do you think this cake is for an adult or child? How do you know?

Narrative/Expository
The SLP's IDEA Companion

6. Leila put down the quilt she was sewing. Her hands were hurting very badly lately, and she needed to take a break. She wanted to finish the quilt by winter, but she had a long way to go and the weather was already getting cooler. She would be disappointed if she didn't finish.

   - What do you picture being sewn?
   - Why did Leila put down the quilt?
   - Why might Leila be disappointed?
   - What month do you think it is?

7. The crowd watched the race with excitement as the runners got close to the finish line. There was one runner in the lead with another close behind him. Their arms pumped quickly as they both aimed to be the first to touch the red ribbon.

   - What is the mood of the crowd?
   - What movement do you picture in this scene?
   - What color do you picture for the ribbon?
   - What might the runners be wearing?

8. The brown and white puppy whimpered as she tried to climb out of the cardboard box. She jumped up onto the side, but slid back down. Her brothers and sisters lay sleeping on an old blue blanket, not noticing their restless sister.

   - What color do you picture the puppy?
   - What movement do you picture in this scene?
   - How is the puppy feeling?
   - Why do you think the puppy wants to get out of the box?

9. The pat of butter dropped into the round, black pan. As it melted, it started to sizzle and bubble. The butter turned from yellow to golden brown as it got hotter.

   - What sound is in this scene?
   - What color do you picture for the pan?
   - What other colors do you picture?
   - What shape do you picture the piece of butter?

10. The huge mountain was covered with fresh snow. The sun shone from straight overhead on the white powder, creating a bright glare. The branches on the evergreen trees hung low with the weight of the snow. The air was silent and calm.

    - What time of day is it?
    - What colors do you picture?
    - What is the mood of this scene?
    - What might have happened the day before?

Benchmark 4: The student identifies the referents of pronouns.

> **Baseline 4:** Have the student follow along as you read these sentences.
>
> 1. The Chinese were responsible for creating the compass, which is used by explorers around the world. **They** discovered that iron ore points north when placed in water. Who does the word *they* refer to?
>
> 2. I like all country music, but the songs **that** are played on 101.7 are my favorite. What does the word *that* refer to?
>
> 3. When Melinda goes to Paige's house for dinner, she always washes **her** hands before she eats. Who washes her hands?
>
> 4. Hundreds of people gathered to meet the soccer team's plane. **They** had watched the game on TV and wanted to congratulate the players. Who watched the game?
>
> 5. The ship's captain told the passenger that **his** life vest was in the cabin. Whose life vest was in the cabin?
>
> 6. Every book in the library belongs to the school, but the book **that** is on the table is Zac's. What does the word *that* refer to?
>
> 7. The woman **who** called sent flowers and the woman **who** came over yesterday baked a cake. Which woman sent flowers?
>
> 8. The sun shone on the flower as **its** petals opened. What does the word *its* refer to?
>
> 9. The lion and tiger, **which** the students saw at the zoo, were named Felix and Hans. What does the word *which* refer to?
>
> 10. Evan's mom surprised a burglar in her apartment when she came home from work. Luckily **he** quickly ran out the door. Who does the word *he* refer to?

Benchmark 5: The student identifies concrete and inferential questions in text.

> **Baseline 5:** Ask the student, "What kind of information do you need to answer this question?"
>
> > *Note:* The words *concrete* and *inferential* may be replaced by the vocabulary you used in therapy to indicate the type of text questions. Answers are in parentheses.

1. When did WWI start? (concrete)

2. How is your school like ones in the early 1900s? (inferential)

3. What are the differences between a topographic and political map? (concrete)

4. What shape are the holes in a wax honeycomb? (concrete)

5. If you were able to talk to Abraham Lincoln, what would you say? (inferential)

6. What methods do historians use to learn about the past? (concrete)

7. What is pottery made of? (concrete)

8. Who was the first king of Babylon? (concrete)

9. How did the Egyptians dress compared to how we dress today? (inferential)

10. Compare the voyage routes of Magellan and Columbus. (concrete)

Goal: to improve the understanding and use of the language of classroom material at the 5th/6th grade levels

Benchmark 1: The student identifies elements of story grammar including internal responses of characters.

Baseline 1: Using a story from the 5th/6th grade curriculum, ask the student:

What was _____'s problem?
How did he/she try to solve it?
What other ways might the character have tried to solve the problem?
What do other characters in the story think about what he/she is doing to solve the problem?
How does the plan work? Does _____ achieve the goal?
How does _____ feel at the end? Why?
How do the other characters feel at the end? Do they feel differently than they did before they knew _____'s plan? If so, why?

Benchmark 2: The student draws inferences from narrative material.

Baseline 2: Using a story from the 5th/6th grade curriculum, ask the student about information requiring an inference. For example, take a passage such as "Exhausted from working a 10-hour shift in the iron mine, Warren dragged himself up the stairs to his bedroom."

Questions:
Will Warren have a hard time falling asleep?
How do you think Warren feels about going to work the next morning?
Do you think Warren was used to working so long?

Benchmark 3: The student creates a "character sketch" describing main attributes of a developed character.

Baseline 3: Have the student choose a character from the story, identify three features which have been clearly explored (e.g., how the character *looks*: hair color, build, way of dressing; how the character *acts*: attitude, disposition; and what the character *does*: hobbies, talents, job, sports), and create several sentences about each topic area.

Judge the accuracy by:

- inclusion of a topic sentence
- cohesion (Is the use of pronouns clear?)
- sequence (Does the order of sentences make sense?)
- topic maintenance (Do the ideas fit the correct topic?)

Benchmark 4: The student compares and contrasts main characters in a story.

Baseline 4: Have the student choose two characters (e.g., protagonist and antagonist). Say, "Tell me about the two main characters in the story. Explain how they are alike and different." Judge accuracy by:

- clear explanation of roles, including how roles contribute to the problem of the story line (e.g., They both want to win the science fair contest.)
- defining features of characters, including similarities (e.g., personality, background, likes/dislikes, goals)
- deciphering reasons one "wins" out over the other, how the winning character's persona contributes to the solving of the problem (e.g., determination, dishonesty, kindness), and how each character reacts to the outcome (e.g., disappointment, anger, resentment, pride, pleasure)

> **Goal:** to improve the understanding and use of the language of classroom material at the 7th – 12th grade levels

Benchmark 1: The student interprets concrete and implied meanings of text.

> **Baseline 1:** Using curricular text, have the student identify events, characters, and ideas in a story that have implied meaning.
>
> For example ask, "What is *The Tortoise and the Hare* a reference to?" (a virtue)
>
> [Other examples: *East of Eden* (a historical event), *Animal Farm* (government), "The Road Less Taken" (a philosophy)]
>
> "How do the personalities of the characters in the story reflect that connection?" (The tortoise is determined — tries to reach his goal even though it looks like there is no way he will win. The hare is overly confident, bragging about his speed and ability.)
>
> "What point is the author trying to make?" (If a person is dedicated to doing something, he can overcome odds that may seem impossible.)
>
> "How does this story apply to today's culture?" (It gives us confidence when we come across tasks that are beyond what we think we can do.)

Benchmark 2: The student organizes information using SQ3R (survey, question, read, review, report) and outlining.

> **Baseline 2:** Have the student use SQ3R and outlining to organize information for tasks required in class.
>
> Possible Tasks:
> - story retelling (book reports)
> - factual retelling (summarizing)
> - fictional stories or guided stories (usually mirrors a theme)
> - expositions (on how to do something)
> - descriptions (of a thing or place)
> - reporting (as a reporter)
> - persuasive pieces (convince someone of something)
> - business letters
> - friendly letters

Measure for:

- providing important details (Does the student include the main points?)
- using colorful, clear vocabulary (Does the student use original words or only those from the text?)
- relating one idea to the next (Is the sequence logical?)
- demonstrating reasoning as for a logical argument (Is the argument supported by facts?)
- using appropriate language for audience ("formal" vs. "casual")

Benchmark 3: The student recognizes and interprets persuasion techniques (e.g., promises, dares, flattery) in media messages.

Baseline 3: Read the following ad slogans to the student. Ask questions like:

   a. What is the message?
   b. What do you think the advertisers might be selling?
   c. What kind of technique are they using to get you to buy their product?
   d. How is the slogan trying to make you feel about yourself?
   e. Why is this a ploy?

1. Push the limit.
   a) be extreme; b) might be a car; c) dare; d) need to be better; e) I may get in trouble or break laws.

2. Power is nothing without control.
   a) It doesn't matter if I just have something powerful, I have to be able to control it; b) stereo speakers, brakes on a bike, video game controller; c) promise; d) what I have is worthless compared to this new item; e) It makes me want to buy something I might not need.

3. Lead the herd.
   a) be the first/the leader; b) new type of clothing, new sport; c) promise; d) I deserve to be the first to have what everyone else will want; e) It may not be something I really want to have or do.

4. Shred the competition.
   a) be the best; b) sports equipment; c) promise; d) I need to be better at this activity. If I buy it, I will be much better than everyone else; e) Just having this product won't make me that much better.

5. the choice of champions
   a) If I am a champion, I will buy this product; b) food, shoes; c) flattery; d) Since I am a champion, I need this product; e) This product won't make me into a champion.

6. time to get serious
   a) until now I haven't been serious enough; b) study tool, test preparation manual;
   c) dare/challenge; d) I need to quit goofing off; e) I can be serious about/dedicated to
   something without this product.

7. when only the best will do
   a) Anything else is less than the best; b) personal care products (make-up, shampoo);
   c) flattery; d) I deserve the best for myself; e) This product won't make me better.

8. Play to win.
   a) The most important thing is winning; b) equipment to help me play better; c) dare
   or promise; d) It's not worth playing unless I win; e) Not everyone can win even if
   they all use this product. It's okay to play just for fun.

9. smart ideas for a stupid world
   a) People who use this product are smart; b) something like computers; c) flattery;
   d) I need to use this product to show that I'm smarter than everyone else; e) A product
   alone can't make me smarter.

10. Do you have what it takes?
    a) Prove that you can do it; b) clothing, sports drink; c) dare; d) I can compete
    because of what I wear/drink/own; e) This product alone can't help me compete that
    much better.

Benchmark 4: The student distinguishes between fact and opinion.

Baseline 4: Read the following sentences. Have the student determine if they are fact or
fiction.

1. Algebra is the branch of mathematics in which letters are used to
   represent basic arithmetic relations. (fact)

2. An acquittal (i.e., when the jury decides that the defendant is not guilty)
   happens too often in our courts. (opinion)

3. The Romans named the days of the week in honor of the sun, moon, and
   various planets. (fact)

4. Ambulances drawn by horses were first used in the 1850s during the
   Crimean War. (fact)

5. The bass part of a quartet is the easiest part to sing. (opinion)

6. No one wants to go to the islands of the Arctic Ocean because of all the
   ice. (opinion)

7. The avocado contains 10-20 percent oil and is rich in protein. (fact)

8. Jack Russell Terriers, which are known for their high energy, are the best dogs to own. (opinion)

9. Badlands National Park has a wildlife population that includes bighorn sheep and antelope. (fact)

10. Captain Cook, a famous British explorer who was killed in the Hawaiian Islands, made a foolish mistake by returning there. (opinion)

Oral-Motor/Articulation

Clear speech is an intricate part of the listening and speaking curriculum. It is important that students use intelligible speech to share their knowledge and opinions. Often students who have difficulty communicating clearly in the classroom also have difficulty with phonological awareness and word attack skills. If the student's auditory discrimination is poor, phonics and spelling suffers. In terms of socialization, these students may be reluctant to participate in class discussions and may have poor interactions with peers.

The benchmarks in this unit are divided into several components: Oral-Motor Skills, Articulation Skills, and Student/Parent/Teacher Involvement. The Oral-Motor section focuses on differentiation, strengthening, and endurance conditioning of the tongue. This section also gives guidelines for measuring lateral margin stabilization which is required for accurate production of almost all sounds (Boshart, 1997). The Articulation Skills section outlines the hierarchy of articulation complexity. The format accommodates both the single sound approach and the phonological process approach. It allows you to specify a single sound or class of sounds and follow the hierarchy needed to achieve automaticity. The Student/Parent/Teacher Involvement section gives suggestions for writing benchmarks that put responsibility on the student and other adults with whom the student spends time. This is especially useful during the carryover stage of therapy.

Classroom materials should be used whenever possible as stimuli for speech practice. For example, you can use reading text at all grades and/or levels, either to identify pictures that have the target sound, name and describe pictures, read the text, or discuss what was read. As the targets in this section will vary greatly from student to student, specific baselines of each level are not given. Therapy notes are the best source for determining to which degree a benchmark has been met.

Oral-Motor/Articulation

Oral-Motor Skills

Goal: to improve effective communication in the classroom by increasing intelligibility through oral-motor strengthening

Benchmark 1: The student achieves independent movement of the tongue from lips and teeth by performing movements on command.

    Baseline 1: Instruct the student to perform the following tasks:

- protrude the tongue without contact with lips or teeth
- move the tongue laterally from corner to corner of the mouth without touching the teeth or lips

Benchmark 2: The student achieves independent movement of the back of the tongue from the tongue tip by performing movements on command.

    Baseline 2: Instruct the student to lift the back of the tongue as if to produce the phoneme /k/, but without sound.

Benchmark 3: The student achieves independent movement of the tongue tip from the tongue body by performing movements on command.

    Baseline 3: Instruct the student to lift the tongue tip from the floor of the mouth to the alveolar ridge while keeping the body of the tongue flat and without jaw movement.

Benchmark 4: The student achieves independent movement of the tongue tip from the jaw by performing movements on command.

    Baseline 4: Instruct the student to produce tongue clicks without jaw movement (i.e., keeping sides of tongue pressed against inside of upper back teeth and only moving the tongue tip to "click").

Benchmark 5: The student achieves lateral margin stabilization of the tongue.

    Baseline 5: Instruct the student to:

- hold the sides of the tongue against the inside of the back teeth
- pull the tongue back with the sides pressed against the back molars without lifting the tongue tip (i.e., won't see the bottom of the tongue)

> **Goal:** to improve effective communication in the classroom by increasing intelligibility through sound discrimination and sound production practice

Benchmark 1: The student achieves meaningful contrast of the target sound/structure and his production of the target by distinguishing pictures of both.

> *Note:* This and subsequent benchmarks refer to the target production as *sound* or *structure*. *Sound* indicates the phoneme (e.g., /r/, /s/, /l/) in error, while *structure* indicates the group of sounds (e.g., blends, final consonants, stridents) in error.

Baseline 1: Show the student minimal pair pictures. Have him identify the pictures of the word containing the target and the word containing the errored production.

Benchmark 2: The student produces the target sound in isolation.

Benchmark 3: The student produces the target sound/structure in syllables.

Benchmark 4: The student produces the target sound/structure in words.

Benchmark 5: The student produces the target sound/structure in sentences.

Benchmark 6: The student produces the target sound/structure in structured activities (e.g., picture description, storytelling, reading aloud, greetings) with cues.

Benchmark 7: The student produces the target sound/structure in spontaneous conversation without cues.

Baselines 2-7: Instruct the student to produce the target sound in the appropriate structure. Tally accuracy and compute the percentage.

These benchmarks are best measured by observing progress across therapy sessions. Since targets of remediation vary greatly, lists of sounds, syllables, sentences, etc. are not listed here. Materials from the classroom curriculum are a great source of baseline stimulus at all levels. Commercial materials designed to target specific sounds and structures are widely available (e.g., *SPARC Revised, SPARC R, SPARC S, SPARC L, Phonology for Groups: Thematic Activities for Everyday Settings, Webber's Jumbo Articulation Drill Book,* and *"Say and Do" Mazes for Articulation*)[1].

[1]See References, pages 160 – 162, for complete bibliographical information.

Student/Parent/Teacher Involvement

Benchmark 1: The student returns speech homework with parent's signature indicating completion.

    Baseline 1: Measure this benchmark by using the therapy log to determine if the student has consistently returned homework during reporting time.

Benchmark 2: The teacher provides cues as directed by the clinician to facilitate carryover to classroom activities several times daily.

    Baseline 2: Use teacher report to measure this benchmark. You may want to establish a written communication system with the teacher to make sure this happens.

Benchmark 3: The student demonstrates use of the new speech skill ten times a week and takes responsibility for speech progress by keeping a journal/log of when speech skill was used.

    Baseline 3: Check the student's speech journal on a regular basis. It may be helpful to have columns designated for the day and time, the name of the person to whom the student speaks, and the initials of that person.

Date	Time	Used new sound to . . .	Initials
9/18	5:00	*ask Mom to go out to play*	*SL*

Benchmark 4: The parent provides opportunities for the student to use the new speech skills at home as directed by the clinician and measured by parent report.

    Baseline 4: Once the student is able to produce the sound in sentences (or when appropriate), encourage the parent to provide times during the day when the student can specifically focus on speech skills (e.g., while looking at a book, during dinnertime talking, while explaining the school day's activities).

Phonological Awareness

Phonological awareness is the ability to make distinctions in auditory stimuli. It includes the skills of rhyming and alliteration as well as the ability to segment sentences, syllables, and words. It can be thought of as the ability to divide the "whole" into "parts." Phonological awareness draws on metalinguistic skills to manipulate sounds and recognize similarities and differences between the units of language. Early evidence of these skills are observed in young children who enjoy hearing repetitive patterns of language, creating rhymes, and discovering words that have the same sounds as in their names.

Children who are slow to acquire language or speech may also have difficulty with phonological awareness. Those children with early speech and language problems characterized by difficulty differentiating similar sounding words, recognizing word boundaries, producing words with complex sound clusters, and performing rapid naming tasks will most likely have problems with reading readiness skills. As speech-language pathologists with expertise in phonological structures, we have an opportunity to affect the educational future for these children. Phonological awareness skills must be in place before meaningful correlations between sounds and symbols (i.e., letters) can be made (Goldsworthy, 1999).

Left untreated, weak phonological awareness skills do not resolve themselves. Students in the secondary grades still struggling in this area have spelling problems and are left without strategies to decipher unfamiliar words. Both reading fluency and comprehension suffer.

Because the general education curriculum targets foundational skills such as phonological awareness and phonics instruction in the kindergarten, first, and second grades, the baselines and benchmarks in this unit focus on these grades. For students beyond this level, you can use these same baselines and benchmarks as long as you adjust the vocabulary to the appropriate level of curriculum or area of interest.

Phonological Awareness

K - 2nd Grade

> **Goal:** to improve the perception of phoneme relationships in order to facilitate decoding skills

Benchmark 1: When given a word, the student creates a rhyming word.

> *Note:* Accept nonsense words as evidence of the target skill.

> **Baseline 1:** Say to the student, "Tell me a word that rhymes with _____."

blue	table
stop	puddle
rope	terrible
flower	banister
yellow	carrier

Benchmark 2: The student segments a multi-syllabic word into syllables.

> **Baseline 2:** Say to the student: "Tell me how many syllables you hear in the word I say."

2 Syllables	*3 Syllables*	*4 Syllables*	*5 Syllables*	*6 Syllables*
apple	elephant	helicopter	tyrannosaurus	autobiography
singer	dinosaur	triceratops	hippopotamus	endocrinologist
glasses	basketball	emergency	pediatrician	cardiovascular
farmer	Saturday	motorcycle	microprocessor	transdisciplinary
coffee	computer	rhinoceros	refrigerator	anti-establishment

Benchmark 3: The student judges words based on the beginning, middle, and ending sounds.

> **Baselines 3A and 3B:** Follow the prompts below and on the next page. Note that there is both a receptive (A) and expressive (B) component to the baseline.

Baseline 3A

Beginning Sounds
1. Tell me if the word I say begins with the sound /b/.
   big   *better*   prop   clip   *back*

2. Tell me if the word I say begins with the sound /s/.
   dogs *snake* hush *sleep* glass

3. Tell me if the word I say begins with the sound /ee/.
   eagle smart egg tree *eat*

4. Tell me if the word I say begins with the sound /n/.
   orange *never* him *not* phone

5. Tell me if the word I say begins with the sound /dʒ/.
   bridge *jump* chick beige *jacks*

Middle Sounds

1. Tell me if the word I say has the sound /ā/ in the middle.
   cape sat tie *same* aimed

2. Tell me if the word I say has the sound /ĭ/ in the middle.
   put *sit* keep *swish* mix

3. Tell me if the word I say has the sound /oo/ in the middle.
   shoot boat book *blue* cup

4. Tell me if the word I say has the sound /ɜ/ in the middle.
   hurt run *firm* *shirt* ripe

5. Tell me if the word I say has the sound /ĕ/ in the middle.
   bed milk *smell* feel *neck*

Ending Sounds

1. Tell me if the word I say ends with the sound /n/.
   can champ nose *tin* cheep

2. Tell me if the word I say ends with the sound /sh/.
   mint cheese *fish* *radish* wake

3. Tell me if the word I say ends with the sound /oo/.
   shoe boy up eat *view*

4. Tell me if the word I say ends with the sound /v/.
   van *cave* phone *of* *leave*

5. Tell me if the word I say ends with the sound /t/.
   hot tell bed *spot* *bat*

Baseline 3B: Say to the student, "Listen to these two words. Tell me how they sound the same."

1. hop - keep	6. sky - sail
2. milk - man	7. flip - few
3. ski - me	8. drink - dump
4. pool - sell	9. white - when
5. cup - cow	10. man - in

Benchmark 4: The student segments words into phonemes.

Baseline 4: Say to the student, "How many sounds do you hear in the word _____?"

CV (2):	toe	see	shoe	buy	key
VC (2):	eel	eat	off	edge	ape
CVC (3):	chief	cape	ship	bill	tote
CCVC (4):	black	spot	break	green	crate
CVCC (4):	books	milk	find	pitched	pint
CCVCC (5):	floods	scold	grapes	crisp	spent

Benchmark 5: The student adds, subtracts, and substitutes phonemes in words to create new words.

Baseline 5: Ask the student, "What word could you make if you _____?"

add /k/ to the beginning of *lean* (clean)
add /t/ to the beginning of *ray* (tray)
add /s/ to the beginning of *cool* (school)
add /d/ to the beginning of *rink* (drink)

add /t/ to the end of *star* (start)
add /s/ to the end of *how* (house)
add /m/ to the end of *are* (arm)
add /th/ to the end of *true* (truth)
add /l/ to the end of *too* (tool)

take away the /m/ in *mat* (at)
take away the /r/ in *bread* (bed)
take away the /k/ in *scope* (soap)
take away the /p/ in *plate* (late)
take away the /h/ in *heat* (eat)

take away the /d/ in *seed* (see)
take away the /t/ in *note* (no)
take away the /m/ in *farm* (far)
take away the /ch/ in *arch* (are)
take away the /s/ in *scream* (cream)

"What word can you make if you take the word _____?"

cat and take away the /t/ and replace it with /b/ (cab)
scare and take away the /k/ and replace it with /t/ (stare)
bench and take away the /ch/ and replace it with /d/ (bend)
glass and take away the /l/ and replace it with /r/ (grass)
dog and take away the /ŏ/ and replace it with /ĭ/ (dig)

Benchmark 6:   The student blends isolated sounds together.

Baseline 6:   Say to the student, "Listen to these sounds. Put them together to make a word."

CV:	s - aw	k - ey	sh - ow
VC:	e - gg	a - t(e)	u - p
CVC:	w - e - t	l - oo - k	ch - o - p
CCVC:	c - l - a - ss	s - p - ee - ch	t - r - i - p
CVCC:	s - o - l - v(e)	th - i - n - k	p - ai - n - t
CCVCC:	p - l - a - t(e) - s	g - r - a - p(e) - s	t - r - i- c(ke) - d

Pragmatics

The ability to use language for a purpose is essential for a student to function in the social realm of education. While the focus of classroom instruction is academic, a "hidden curriculum" also exists. In order for a student to be successful in the classroom, she must know the rules of classroom behavior: waiting for her turn, raising her hand, standing correctly in line, sharing common space, working on a team project, and addressing her teacher with appropriate language, just to name a few. In addition to the classroom, she needs to know playground expectancies as well as how to make and maintain friendships.

When pragmatics is an area of deficit, social skills suffer. In the early grades, this communication problem causes confusion with conversation rules. The student this affects makes irrelevant, out-of-place comments and off-topic remarks. Nonverbal communication cues are not considered and rules of personal space are disregarded. The ability to adjust one's language according to the situation is weak.

As the social scene intensifies at the secondary level, so do pragmatic demands. Adults and adolescents are far less tolerant of the pragmatic errors that may have once been considered cute in a young child. Phone conversations, dating rituals, teenage slang vocabulary, multiple teachers' styles, and just "hanging out" present new challenges of social skills for the adolescent. Consequently, students with pragmatic problems have a hard time fitting in, often acting out aggressively in frustration.

Because this area of language has fewer boundaries of skill expectancies based on grade, the benchmarks are divided into elementary (K-6) and secondary (7-12) levels. These are strictly guidelines. Your clinical judgment and feedback from the teacher are necessary in knowing which skills are needed for each particular student. Furthermore, because pragmatics are difficult to measure as an isolated skill, the baselines combined with teacher/parent input should be considered in assessing the carryover of a new pragmatic skill.

Pragmatics

K - 6th Grade

> **Goal:** to adapt or change oral language to fit the situation by following the rules of conversation with peers and adults

Benchmark 1: The student adjusts his language during a role-playing situation according to an audience.

Baseline 1: Say to the student, "We're going to practice our communication skills. Let's role-play a situation."

> *Note:* The following are examples of ways language is adjusted. The type of skill can be specified in the benchmark or serve as a general guide to meeting the benchmark.
>
> a) Polite
> b) Persuade
> c) Urgency
> d) Tact
> e) Topic Maintenance
> f) Defense
> g) Vocal Intensity

a) Polite
"What would you say/how would you act if _____?"

1. you want to use the telephone in the office to call home
2. you need to borrow a quarter from an adult
3. you want a refill for your soda at a restaurant
4. you want to find out if you made the soccer team
5. you didn't understand an assignment and want to ask your teacher
6. you need to talk to someone who is talking with someone else
7. you need help finding a book in the library
8. you want to find out the price of a toy
9. you need directions to someone's house
10. you need to find out what time a movie starts

b) Persuade
"What would you say/how would you act if you were trying to persuade _____?"

1. your parents to let you stay up late
2. your teacher to change a bad grade on a test

3. your grandpa to buy your favorite cereal
4. your brother to let you borrow his bike
5. your best friend to tell you a secret
6. your mom to give you a ride to the mall
7. your neighbor to take care of your cat for the weekend
8. the librarian to waive the fine for an overdue book
9. your teacher to let the class have a longer recess
10. your neighbor to buy cookies that you're selling for school

c) Urgency
"What would you say/how would you act if _____?"

1. a student fell on the playground
2. your friend was sick in the bathroom
3. you saw an accident on your way home from school
4. smoke was coming from the oven, and your mom wasn't in the room
5. the bathtub was overflowing with water
6. your two-year-old sister broke a glass vase
7. you accidentally threw your retainer in the trash after lunch
8. you spilled red punch on your shirt
9. you got stung by a bee
10. you fell out of a boat and couldn't swim

d) Tact
"What would you say/how would you act if _____?"

1. you want to tell your friend her/his shirt is on backward
2. you suspect someone you know is having a baby, and the person hasn't told you
3. you need to tell a classmate not to copy from your test paper
4. you need to let someone know you can't go to his/her birthday party
5. you need to tell a friend he/she has food in his/her teeth
6. you want to apologize for being rude or mean
7. you want to find out why a classmate has missed a week of school
8. you found out your teacher was getting married
9. your friend's grandma died
10. your friend won the game you were playing together

e) Topic Maintenance
"We're going to talk about _____. I'll start."
> *Note:* The target number of exchanges (e.g., three turns each) is at the discretion of the clinician.

1. our favorite foods
2. things we like to do over the summer
3. a game that we really like
4. our favorite sport

5. the last book we read
6. why we like our friends
7. our favorite restaurant
8. the last movie we saw
9. our favorite family activities
10. what we would like to learn how to do

f) Defense
"What would you say/how would you act if _____?"

1. your teacher accused you of cheating on a test
2. a kid on the playground embarrassed you by teasing you
3. the cashier at the grocery store accused you of stealing a candy bar
4. your mom punished you for something your sister did
5. another student pushed your friend and blamed you
6. you borrowed a comic book from your friend, and your dog ripped it up
7. someone teased your best friend
8. you got home too late last night to do homework, and your teacher wants to know where it is
9. a dollar is missing from a classmate's desk, and the teacher asks you if you took it
10. you signed your parent's name on your speech homework, and the speech-language pathologist asks you about it

g) Vocal Intensity
"Show me the right kind of voice to use when _____."

1. you need to ask the person next to you to borrow an eraser
2. you need to tell the attendant across the playground that someone fell off the monkey bars
3. you are in a movie theater when the movie is about to start, and you want your stepdad to pass the popcorn
4. you have forgotten a student's name who is new to your class, and you want to ask another classmate without the new student overhearing
5 you want to ask your teacher, who is sitting across from you, if you can use the rest room
6. you want to tell a friend (so that no one else will hear) that her shirt is ripped
7. you need to tell your mom, who is upstairs, that the laundry is finished
8. you want to get the attention of the students in your classroom when it is somewhat noisy
9. you want to tell your teacher in confidence that you don't feel very well and would like to go to the nurse's office
10. you are in a library, and you need to ask the librarian to help you find a book

Benchmark 2: The student asks for specific clarification when the message is unclear.

   Baseline 2:   Follow the prompts provided.

> *Note:* Some types of unclear messages are ones that are muddled; have an unfamiliar word; have directions given too soft or too fast; or have inexplicit, ambiguous, or complex directions. The goal of this activity is to measure the student's ability to pinpoint what he has missed regardless of any interference to the message. Materials can be simply a blank sheet of paper and a pencil. Directions are intentionally simple to isolate a pragmatic skill from that of vocabulary.

1. Use a normal rate and volume as you say, "Write your name in a corner of the paper."
    Target: correct response

2. Use a muffled, almost inaudible voice as you say the location of the circle, "Draw a circle in the middle of the page."
    Target: clarification of where

3. Use a normal rate and volume as you say, "Put a star at the pintar of the paper."
    Target: clarification of word meaning

4. Use a rate of speech that is too fast to understand as you say, "Draw a line under your name."
    Target: clarification of what to do

5. Use a normal rate and volume as you say, "Put a crescent-shaped square around the circle."
    Target: I don't understand or I can't, etc.

6. Use a muffled, almost inaudible voice as you say, "Draw a heart at the bottom of the page."
    Target: clarification of what to do

7. Use a normal rate and volume as you say, "In the middle of the heart, mitigate a caliper."
    Target: clarification of word meaning

8. Use a rate of speech that is too fast to understand as you say the location part of the direction, "Draw a square next to the heart."
    Target: clarification of location

9. Use a normal rate and volume as you say, "Draw an arrow pointing up, anywhere on the page."
    Target: correct response

10. Use a normal rate and volume as you say, "Put a big dot on the facade of the arrow."
    Target: clarification of word meaning

> **Goal:** to adapt or change oral language to fit the situation by following the rules of conversation with peers and adults

Benchmark 1: The student keeps a journal of slang terms or idiomatic language and its context heard from other students, explains the meanings, and demonstrates appropriate use in role-play situations.

> *Note:* A specified number (e.g., 10 entries per quarter) can give the student additional structure as well as more responsibility to meet this benchmark.

Baseline 1: Determine if the journal has the specified number of entries. Ask the following questions about the situation:

1. What do you know about the conversation that was going on?
2. What other words were used in the same sentence?
3. Why do you think the speaker used the word/phrase _____?
4. Let's set up a different situation in which you might use this phrase/word.

Example: The student makes a journal entry of the phrase "yard sale."
Clinician: "What do you know about the conversation?"
Student: "I know the speaker was talking about a recent ski trip."
Clinician: "What was the context of (or what other words were used with) the new word?"
Student: "The speaker said, 'It was a total yard sale when I lost my balance.'"
Clinician: "So what do you think happened when he lost his balance?"
Student: "He probably fell pretty bad."
Clinician: "Why do you think he used the phrase 'yard sale'?"
Student: "It was like his stuff was all over: his poles, his skis, his cap – like when you have a yard sale, stuff is lying around all over."
Clinician: "Tell me another situation in which you might use that phrase."

Benchmark 2: The student demonstrates negotiation skills by describing and resolving conflict in a role-play situation.

Baseline 2: Ask the student, "How would you handle a situation in which _____?"

1. your friend borrowed a brand-new book from you and returned it with pages torn
2. you had an argument with a friend, and then he didn't invite you to his birthday party

3. your family is going on vacation and you are allowed to bring along two friends. You know another friend's feelings will be hurt when he/she finds out you didn't choose him/her.
4. someone in your class asks you to lie for him/her if the teacher asks you if he/she cheated (even though you saw him/her do it)
5. you found out that a classmate was spreading false rumors about you
6. you had several people over to your house to study, and the next day you discover $20 missing from your room
7. you know your friend's boyfriend is going out with another girl
8. you are at a party where some kids are drinking alcohol, and some of your classmates are pressuring you to drink
9. you need to get a ride from a classmate, but there are more people in the car than there are seat belts
10. your older sister was out past her curfew, and she asks you not to tell your parents

Semantics

A strong base in semantics is essential for survival in school. Having the ability to judge information and incorporate it into what is already known is the foundation for learning. Children for whom this is difficult have trouble academically. Even kindergarten requires the skills of relating experiences, participating in class discussion, answering questions, and grasping new concepts presented on a daily basis. When students at this age have deficits in semantics, they miss the structure upon which future comprehension is built.

As students progress through school, they are expected to grasp information increasingly less concrete in nature. Idioms, metaphors, and implicit meanings of text cause much difficulty for the student with language learning difficulties in the upper and advanced grades. The common thread of comprehending information and pragmatic self-expression is woven throughout the academic curriculum.

The baselines in this section are written for easy administration. Most baselines have clear-cut answers, but some will require clinical judgment. For the baselines written in paragraph form, the questions following each paragraph correspond to a certain benchmark. Only the questions pertaining to the targeted benchmark need be administered. Specific guidelines and suggestions are provided in the form of "notes" throughout this section.

Semantics

Kindergarten

Goal: to improve the understanding and use of the language used in classroom material at the K grade level

Benchmark 1: The student classifies items by category and explains their relationships.

    Baseline 1: Using the pictures on pages 135 – 136, have the student find the picture that does not belong in each group and tell why.

Benchmark 2: The student identifies basic opposites involving direction, attribute, and function.

    Baseline 2: Have the student give an opposite for each word below.

        hot (cold)
        big (little, small)
        up (down)
        behind (in front)
        last (first)
        good (bad)
        tall (short, little)
        inside (outside)
        take (give)
        happy (sad, unhappy)

Benchmark 3: The student interprets pictures to identify cause-effect.

    Baseline 3: Using the pictures on pages 137 – 138, have the student identify the problem and why it might have happened. Judge the benchmark as met if the student identifies the relationship between an action and a consequence.

Benchmark 4: The student interprets pictures to predict logical outcomes.

    Baseline 4: Using the pictures on pages 139 – 140, ask the student, "What would happen if _____?"

> **Goal:** to improve the understanding and use of the language used in classroom material at the 1st/2nd grade levels

Benchmark 1: The student indicates the main idea of a paragraph.

> **Baseline 1:** With the student following along, read the baseline sentences and ask the corresponding questions.
>
> > *Note:* Since text was probably used to practice this benchmark in the therapy session, it would benefit the student to be able to see the words in print as well as hear them read. Use your clinical judgment in deciding whether or not to use the multiple-choice format provided.

1. Kyle was painting a picture for a school project. He only had blue and yellow so he mixed them together to make green.

   What is the main idea?
   a. Blue and yellow make green (mixing colors).
   b. Kyle has yellow paint.
   c. Kyle is a messy painter.

2. Keisha felt sad because her best friend, Maggie, had moved to another town several weeks ago. She was lonely without her. Just then, her mom handed her a letter. It was from Maggie! Keisha ran inside to read the letter.

   What is the main idea?
   a. Keisha had friends to play with.
   b. Keisha got a letter that made her feel better.
   c. Keisha lost the letter.

3. Michael watched as his dad mowed the lawn, trimmed the bushes, and pulled the weeds.

   What is the main idea?
   a. The yard was a mess.
   b. Michael wanted to play football.
   c. Dad did yard work.

4. Chelsea's balloon floated up in the air and she began to cry. Her brother Zach ran to get it. It had gotten stuck in a tree. Zach got it and gave it back to Chelsea. "Next time, don't let go," said Zach.

   What is the main idea?
   a. Chelsea began to cry.
   b. Zach gets the balloon.
   c. The balloon stays in the tree.

5. Whitney left the kitchen after baking cupcakes. When she came back, she couldn't find the cupcakes. Then she looked at her dog, Buddy. There was some cake on the dog's nose. " I can't find the cupcakes," said Whitney, "but I think I know where they went!"

   What is the main idea?
   a. Whitney ate cupcakes.
   b. Buddy made a cupcake.
   c. Whitney knew where the cupcakes went.

6. "We'll have to have our picnic in the car," Kim's mom said. "It's starting to rain. Why don't we take all the food to the car and eat it in there? Maybe the rain will stop soon."

   What is the main idea?
   a. There were too many ants.
   b. They forgot the food.
   c. The rain did not stop the picnic.

7. Lorin had just finished raking all the leaves in the yard into a big pile. Suddenly a wind came and scattered the leaves. Lorin tried to stuff as many as he could in a bag, but it was no use. The leaves were all over the yard again.

   What is the main idea?
   a. Lorin wasted his time raking the leaves.
   b. The leaves had been falling all winter.
   c. Rakes are dangerous.

8. April's mom just had a baby boy. April was feeling left out because her new brother was getting all the attention. Her grandpa suggested she help him paint a toy box for the baby. She painted a moon and stars on the box. April felt better because she was doing a job as a big sister.

   What is the main idea?
   a. The baby is cranky.
   b. April is happy the baby is getting attention.
   c. April likes being a big sister.

9. Jacob was playing in the backyard when he found a baby bird on the ground. He looked up to see a nest in the tree above him. He saw that the bird's wing was broken. His mom and he made a small bed for the bird to rest in. In a few weeks, the bird was able to fly again.

   What is the main idea?
   a. Jacob helps a bird.
   b. Jacob breaks his arm.
   c. Birds can't fly.

10. Marcie's mom told her that she couldn't go out to play until she had cleaned her room. Marcie went to her room, but she played with her toys instead. After several hours, Marcie cleaned her room and wanted to go outside. Her mother said it was too late because the sun had already gone down. Marcie was mad.

    What is the main idea?
    a. Marcie's mom was unfair.
    b. Marcie wasted time.
    c. Marcie's room was already clean.

Benchmark 2: The student uses *who, what, where, when, how*, and *why* questions appropriately.

Baseline 2: Use the same format to measure this skill as you did teaching it in therapy. One possibility is a trivia game. This type of setup lends itself to creating questions. Depending on the ability of the student, you may want to provide the target "wh" word. Say to the student, "I'll give you an answer and you make up a question." For example, "The answer is 'behind the desk.' What question might go with that answer?" (Where is the chair?)

1. Target: "Where ____?"
   in the classroom
   on a chair
   under a pillow
   in the ocean
   at the grocery store
   in the refrigerator

2. Target: "When ____?"
   after school
   in July
   tomorrow morning
   yesterday
   2:00 p.m.
   this summer

3. Target: "Who ____?"
   my teacher
   Cinderella
   a mother/father
   a lifeguard
   the principal
   a stranger

4. Target: "How ____?"
   with a spoon
   with some keys
   with a saw
   using your eyes
   with a lawn mower
   with a pencil

5. Target: "Why ____?"
    in case it rains
    because it is cold outside
    so they can see better
    to find out the news
    so you don't get hurt
    to keep our feet dry

6. Target: "What ____?"
    a kitten
    the forest
    the classroom
    a butterfly
    a computer
    a chair

Benchmark 3: The student indicates whether information is real or make-believe (fact or fiction in second grade).

Baseline 3: Ask the student, "If you heard a story about _____, would that be real or make-believe?"

> rabbits that talk (make-believe)
> houses with windows (real)
> candy that was good for you (make-believe)
> letters that needed stamps to be mailed (real)
> buying clothes at the mall (real)
> purple grass (make-believe)
> plants with leaves (real)
> cars that flew in the sky (make-believe)
> cats that went to school (make-believe)
> how milk comes from cows (real)

Benchmark 4: The student gives similarities and differences between two or more related words based on descriptive features (e.g., size, shape, texture, function, color, location, weight).

Baseline 4: Ask the student to tell how each pair is the same and different. Measure accuracy by the number/importance of features (e.g., size, shape, texture, function, color, location, weight).

Pairs	Similarities	Differences
couch and bed	soft; you can lie on them	sit on a couch; sleep on a bed
finger and toe	part of body; ten of each	feet have toes; hands have fingers
bracelet and necklace	jewelry; made out of same material	bracelet around wrist; necklace around neck
cat and tiger	cat family; have whiskers, paws, etc.	cat is house pet; tiger is wild animal
rose and daisy	both are flowers; grow in gardens	rose has thorns; daisy does not; different shape
slippers and shoes	wear on feet	slippers inside; shoes outside
wall and fence	divide land; both tall	wall is solid; you can see through many fences
house and tent	provide shelter	you live in a house; you camp in a tent
banana and strawberry	both fruit; can eat	banana is yellow; strawberry is red
purse and briefcase	hold items needed to carry	purse usually softer, smaller, and like a bag; briefcase shaped like a rectangle

Benchmark 5: The student explains cause and effect relationships.

>**Baseline 5:** Ask the student to give the cause and effect in each situation. Judge the benchmark as met if the student identifies the relationship between an action and a consequence.

1. Sarah was embarrassed when she spilled juice on her white sweater.

2. Michael always gets up really early on his birthday. It's his favorite day of the year.

3. There were so many mosquitoes at camp, we all came home with big bumps on our arms.

4. When the bear got hungry, he went to the stream where there were many fish.

5. Angie was trying to study while her parents had company, so she put cotton in her ears.

6. The bird eggs broke when the wind knocked the nest out of the tree.

7. Tannen tripped on his shoelace and fell to the ground.

8. Amy felt afraid when the electricity went out.

9. Patrice climbed into her grandma's lap to listen to her read a story.

10. His pants were green after he sat on the freshly painted park bench.

Benchmark 6: The student identifies an unknown word in text by brainstorming possible meanings based on context or pictures.

>**Baseline 6:** With the student following along, read the baseline sentences. Ask which word best describes the underlined word.

1. The eyes of a <u>mudskipper</u> can get sunburned if it swims close to the surface.
    A *mudskipper* probably is a: boat
                                           fish
                                           person

2. American Indians painted their faces with bright colors before going into battle. The war paint gave them a scary <u>appearance</u>.
    Appearance probably means: costume
                                              tribe
                                              look

3. In an egg race, each person carries an egg in a spoon for a <u>distance</u> of 15 feet. He then returns and gives the spoon to the next player.
    Distance probably means: how far
                                          the kind of spoon
                                          how fast

4. House mice are not only small, but <u>timid</u>. They won't come out in the open if a person is in the room.
    Timid probably means: brave
                                    shy
                                    ugly

5. The person who works at a lighthouse lives there. He lives in the <u>base</u> of the tower and walks up the stairs to check the light.
    Base probably means: the bottom
                                 the top
                                 outside

6. Some birds live over the water. They often follow ships for days, hoping the sailors will toss <u>scraps</u> of food over the side.
    Scraps probably means: pieces
                                     boards
                                     sand

7. Marsha had many <u>chores</u> to do around the house. She vacuumed the rooms, dusted the furniture, and did the laundry.
    Chores probably means: games
                                   jobs
                                   smells

8. Jenna felt <u>drowsy</u> after a long day at Disneyland. When she got in the car with her family she fell asleep right away.
    Drowsy probably means: excited
                                     angry
                                   tired

9. The little dog looked a little bit <u>odd</u>. He was missing hair in places and had one eye closed.
    Odd probably means: strange
                               happy
                               healthy

10. Mrs. Smith is <u>famous</u> for her oatmeal-raisin cookies. Everyone talks about how wonderful they taste.
    Famous probably means: crooked
                                  well-known
                                  bland

Benchmark 7: The student demonstrates an understanding of math language concepts (e.g., quantity, spatial, ordinal, temporal, operations).

Baseline 7: Measure as described below.

Quantity: Use ten similar items such as blocks, and ask the student to demonstrate the age-appropriate concepts listed below.

First Grade

bigger/smaller (amount) — Have two groups of uneven numbers.
few, some, many, all, half, none
equal amounts

Second Grade

estimation (Have two uneven groups and ask questions like, "Which group is closer to 5?")
more (or greater) than/less than (With two uneven groups, have the student identify each.)
place value (i.e., ones, tens) — Write a double-digit number, and have the student identify it. Write down several double-digit numbers, and ask the student to identify which numbers are in the ones place and which numbers are in the tens place.
single/double digits (Show a series of single- and double-digit numbers, and have the student identify each one.)

Spatial: Use several objects and ask the student to arrange them in a specified relationship to each other.
above/below
under/over
beside
closer or near/farther
first, middle, last
left, right

Ordinal: Place several items in a row and ask the student about their order.
first
second
third
fourth
fifth

Temporal: Ask the questions following each set of concepts.
> longer/shorter
>> "Which is longer, an hour or a day?" (hour)
>> "Which is shorter, a second or a minute?" (second)
> earlier/later
>> "Which comes earlier, morning or evening?" (morning)
>> "Which comes later, 2:00 or 5:00?" (5:00)
> before/after
>> "Which month comes before February?" (January)
>> "What comes after summer?" (fall)

Operations: Read the following math story problems. Have the student determine the operation needed to solve each problem (e.g., "Should you add or subtract?") and what word or words indicate the operation (e.g., "What word/words tell you what to do?").

Addition:
> in all
>> "Jamie put 2 eggs in the cake mix, then put in 2 more. How many eggs were there in all?"
>> "The Red Sox scored 5 runs in the first inning and 2 in the second. How many runs did they have in all by the end of the second inning?"

> total
>> "Five butterflies sat on a branch. Three more joined them. What was the total number of butterflies?"
>> "The park had a slide, swings, and monkey bars. Last week, workers added a teeter-totter and a slide pole. What is the total number of things to play on?"

> all together
>> "Andrea washed 7 paintbrushes after she rinsed 2 sponges. How many tools did she clean all together?"
>> "Tom had a pen, a pencil, and a marker. How many things to write with did he have all together?"

> sum
>> "Kristin threw 5 rocks in the pond. Tony threw in 5 also. What was the sum of the rocks thrown in the pond?"
>> "Lauren helped her stepmom plant daisies, roses, and tulips in the yard. What was the sum of flower types?"

Subtraction:

how many more

"Kelly gave 7 cookies to her friend and kept one for herself. How many more cookies did her friend have?"

"The grocery store down the street has 9 types of cereal. Sue's family buys 3 of them. How many more kinds does the store have that Sue doesn't buy?"

were left

"There were 10 apples on the tree. After I took 5, how many were left?"

"Melody put 8 library books on the counter to check out, but the limit was 5. How many books were left on the counter after she checked out?"

Goal: to improve the understanding and use of the language used in classroom material at the 3rd/4th grade levels

Benchmark 1: The student predicts the content of a passage or story based only on the title or heading.

Benchmark 2: The student identifies the main idea in a paragraph.

Benchmark 3: The student paraphrases a passage by providing three or four important details.

Benchmark 4: The student identifies an unknown word in a sentence.

Benchmark 5: The student predicts the function of an unknown word (action, noun, adjective, etc.).

Benchmark 6: The student predicts the meaning of an unfamiliar word based on context and syntactical cues (e.g., prefix/suffix, root word).

Baselines 1-6: As the student follows along, read the following paragraphs. Ask the questions (1-6) which correspond to the targeted benchmarks.

Note: Although the unfamiliar words in Benchmarks 4, 5, and 6 were taken from 3rd/4th grade curriculum, they may not be unfamiliar to your student. Use your clinical judgment to determine if this skill is emerging as your student encounters novel words in text.

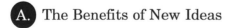 **A.** The Benefits of New Ideas

1. What do you think this paragraph will be about?

An innovation is a new idea or way of doing something. Some innovations really change how we live. They benefit our lives because they help us do something by making it easier, faster, or better. One example of an innovation is the chainsaw. Someone (an innovator) thought a regular saw could be made better by changing it to have many small blades and be powered by a motor instead of a human hand. Innovations tend to improve our lives.

2. In one sentence, what is the main idea of the paragraph?

3. Tell me in your own words what is important in this passage.

4. Look back at the paragraph. Were there any words that were new to you?

5. Look at the word *innovator* in the paragraph. What kind of word is it? Is it a noun, a verb, an adjective, or an adverb?

6. What is an *innovator*?

B. The First Americans

1. What do you think this paragraph will be about?

Many people immigrated to the United States during the 1800s. People saw opportunities to own land, easily find jobs, send their children to good schools, and have freedoms they did not have in their home countries. Thirty million immigrants came to the United States in a 100-year period. This is when people began to call themselves "Americans."

2. In one sentence, what is the main idea of the paragraph?

3. Tell me in your own words what is important in this passage.

4. Look back at the paragraph. Were there any words that were new to you?

5. Look at the word *immigrants* in the paragraph. What kind of word is it? Is it a noun, a verb, an adjective, or an adverb?

6. Who are *immigrants*?

C. Reaching for a Goal in the Sky

1. What do you think this paragraph will be about?

The airplane named the *Voyager* was the first plane to fly around the world without stopping. The plane was very small and lightweight. There were two pilots in the tiny cockpit. The plane flew for 216 hours through strong winds and over tall mountains. Finally the pilots landed at Edwards Air Force Base in California, completing their mission.

2. In one sentence, what is the main idea of the paragraph?

3. Tell me in your own words what is important in this passage.

4. Look back at the paragraph. Were there any words that were new to you?

5. Look at the word *mission* in the paragraph. What kind of word is it? Is it a noun, a verb, an adjective, or an adverb?

6. In this paragraph, what is a *mission*?

D. Making History with Pictures

1. What do you think this paragraph will be about?

The history of the camera is very interesting. The very first camera took eight hours to take a photograph. It took that long for the camera to copy an image onto film. There was a big problem with early photographs, however, because the image faded and disappeared! Then the negative was created so there would be a copy in case the picture disappeared. The camera underwent many more changes before it became what we know it as today.

2. In one sentence, what is the main idea of the paragraph?

3. Tell me in your own words what is important in this passage.

4. Look back at the paragraph. Were there any words that were new to you?

5. Look at the word *negative* in the paragraph. What kind of word is it? Is it a noun, a verb, an adjective, or an adverb?

6. In this paragraph, what does the word *negative* mean?

E. The Wonders of the Brain

1. What do you think this paragraph will be about?

The human brain is an incredible organ. The adult brain weighs only three pounds, yet it can do more than the fastest, most powerful computer. It allows you to make quick decisions, and to see, hear, touch, taste, and even smell. It is the part of your body that controls all of your movements. It lets you remember what you have experienced. If a part of your brain gets damaged, other areas sometimes can be trained to make up for the damaged area.

2. In one sentence, what is the main idea of the paragraph?

3. Tell me in your own words what is important in this passage.

4. Look back at the paragraph. Were there any words that were new to you?

5. Look at the word *incredible* in the paragraph. What kind of word is it? Is it a noun, a verb, an adjective, or an adverb?

6. What does the word *incredible* mean?

F. Facts about Terriers

1. What do you think this paragraph will be about?

There are 24 breeds of terriers. Terriers were originally bred to drive game out of holes in the ground. Most terriers have coarse coats and bushy beards. They are helpful to people by being good watchdogs and by killing household pests like mice and rats.

2. In one sentence, what is the main idea of the paragraph?

3. Tell me in your own words what is important in this passage.

4. Look back at the paragraph. Were there any words that were new to you?

5. Look at the word *game* in the paragraph. What kind of word is it? Is it a noun, a verb, an adjective, or an adverb?

6. What does the word *game* mean?

G. A Popular Place in Delaware

1. What do you think this paragraph will be about?

Wilmington, Delaware, is the only large city in the state. None of the other cities has a population of over 2,000 people. More than two-thirds of the people of Delaware live in the Wilmington metropolitan area, which is located in the far northern part of the state.

2. In one sentence, what is the main idea of the paragraph?

3. Tell me in your own words what is important in this passage.

4. Look back at the paragraph. Were there any words that were new to you?

5. Look at the word *metropolitan* in the paragraph. What kind of word is it? Is it a noun, a verb, an adjective, or an adverb?

6. What does *metropolitan* mean?

H. A Popular Author

1. What do you think this paragraph will be about?

Charles Dickens was a great English novelist and one of the most popular writers of all time. He wrote 20 novels during his life. The common theme in his novels has to do with differences between the attitudes of the poor and rich. He was known for his warmth and humor in writing.

2. In one sentence, what is the main idea of the paragraph?

3. Tell me in your own words what is important in this passage.

4. Look back at the paragraph. Were there any words that were new to you?

5. Look at the word *novelist* in the paragraph. What kind of word is it? Is it a noun, a verb, an adjective, or an adverb?

6. What is a *novelist*?

I. Dolphin Talk

1. What do you think this paragraph will be about?

The communication system of dolphins is very interesting. They communicate with each other by making sounds such as clicks and whistles. Scientists believe that dolphins make different sounds when they are in trouble or when they have found food. Scientists hope to learn more about what all the different sounds mean.

2. In one sentence, what is the main idea of the paragraph?

3. Tell me in your own words what is important in this passage.

4. Look back at the paragraph. Were there any words that were new to you?

5. Look at the word *system* in the paragraph. What kind of word is it? Is it a noun, a verb, an adjective, or an adverb?

6. What does the word *system* mean in this passage?

J. Farm Animal Food

1. What do you think this paragraph will be about?

Hay is a horse and cattle feed made from the dried stems of plants such as grass or oats. After the main part of the plant is removed, the farmer cuts the stems and then bales the hay into big round or square bundles. The bundles of hay are used to feed the farm animals.

2. In one sentence, what is the main idea of the paragraph?

3. Tell me in your own words what is important in this passage.

4. Look back at the paragraph. Were there any words that were new to you?

5. Look at the word *bales* in the paragraph. What kind of word is it? Is it a noun, a verb, an adjective, or an adverb?

6. What does the word *bales* mean in this passage?

Goal: to improve the understanding and use of the language used in classroom material at the 5th/6th grade levels

Benchmark 1: The student will make an inference about a statement read to her.

Baseline 1: With the student following along, read the sentences below. Ask the corresponding inference question. You might want to let the student know that the answer isn't spelled out in the passage.

1. All of his classmates gathered around him, because no one believed he could eat a cake that size.
   What size was the cake?

2. The bell in the hallway rang loudly, signaling the end of class.
   Where did the students go?

3. She pulled her banana out of her lunchbox, disappointed to see that it had rotted.
   What color was the banana?

4. The woman told the passengers to fasten their seat belts and put all their tray tables away.
   Where were they?

5. He proudly sang the "National Anthem" before the umpire started the game.
   Where did this take place?

6. Marcie deposited her first check and thanked the man behind the counter for his help.
   Who was the man?

7. The clock struck twelve as he got home from the party. His parents had already gone to bed.
   What time of day was it?

8. A high-pitched noise filled the air as the red truck left the station.
   Where was the truck going?

9. From the looks of him, one would think he could tear telephone books in half and bend steel bars.
   How did he look?

10. The girl grabbed the warm bread and shoved it in her mouth with big bites.
    Why did the girl eat this way?

Benchmark 2: The student predicts the content of a passage or story based on the title or heading.

Benchmark 3: The student identifies the main idea of a paragraph.

Benchmark 4: The student paraphrases a passage including four important details.

Benchmark 5: The student identifies an unknown word in a sentence.

Benchmark 6: The student predicts the function of an unknown word (e.g., action, noun, adjective).

Benchmark 7: The student brainstorms the meaning of a word based on context and syntactical cues (e.g., prefix/suffix, root word).

Baselines 2-7: As the student follows along, read the following paragraphs. Ask the questions (2-7) which correspond to the targeted benchmarks.

Note: Although the unfamiliar words in Benchmarks 5, 6, and 7 were taken from 5th/6th grade curriculum, they may not be unfamiliar to your student. Use your clinical judgment to determine if this skill is emerging as your student encounters novel words in text.

A. The Danger of Forest Cutting

2. What do you think this passage will be about?

Trees are often cut down and forests cleared in order to build houses or raise crops. This deforestation can create problems such as flooding, the extinction of plants and animals that live there, and the loss of valuable topsoil. This is a problem affecting the whole world and, if not solved, will bring long-term damage to the Earth.

3. In one sentence, what is the main idea in the paragraph?

4. Tell me in your own words what is important in this passage.

5. Look back at the paragraph. Were there any words that were new to you?

6. Look at the word *deforestation* in the paragraph. What kind of word is *deforestation*? Is it a noun, a verb, an adjective, or an adverb?

7. In this passage, what does *deforestation* mean?

B. The Climate of China

2. What do you think this passage will be about?

The climate of China is very diverse. It has many different weather patterns. For example, a cold, dry climate exists in the mountains where very little rain falls, but there is a wet, hot climate along the coast where 80 inches of rain falls a year. More people live near the coast than the mountains.

3. In one sentence, what is the main idea in the paragraph?

4. Tell me in your own words what is important in this passage.

5. Look back at the paragraph. Were there any words that were new to you?

6. Look at the word *diverse* in the paragraph. What kind of word is *diverse*? Is it a noun, a verb, an adjective, or an adverb?

7. What does *diverse* mean in this passage?

C. The Early Days of the Yo-Yo

2. What do you think this passage will be about?

The toy called the "yo-yo" has existed for thousands of years. In 5000 BC the yo-yo was made out of stone and used as a weapon by hunters in the Philippines. The word *yo-yo* means "to return" in a Philippine language. That may explain how it was used. Hunters might have used yo-yos to strike animals from a distance. The hunters could retrieve the yo-yos easily if they missed.

3. In one sentence, what is the main idea in the paragraph?

4. Tell me in your own words what is important in this passage.

5. Look back at the paragraph. Were there any words that were new to you?

6. Look at the word *retrieve* in the paragraph. What kind of word is *retrieve*? Is it a noun, a verb, an adjective, or an adverb?

7. What does *retrieve* mean in this passage?

D. Information from the Past

2. What do you think this passage will be about?

Archeologists use many different sources to find out about the past. One source is artifacts, like coins, tools, and jewelry. These tell us about the lifestyles and customs of people who lived long before us.

3. In one sentence, what is the main idea in the paragraph?

4. Tell me in your own words what is important in this passage.

5. Look back at the paragraph. Were there any words that were new to you?

6. Look at the word *artifacts* in the paragraph. What kind of word is *artifacts*? Is it a noun, a verb, an adjective, or an adverb?

7. What does *artifacts* mean in this passage?

E. Is It a Fact?

2. What do you think this passage will be about?

There are differences between what is considered fact and reasoned judgment. Facts are statements that can be proven or validated in some way. Reasoned judgments can be based on facts, like how something may have come to be, but they haven't been proven. For example, it is a fact that dinosaurs lived on Earth, but how they died is a reasoned judgment. We use both to understand the past.

3. In one sentence, what is the main idea in the paragraph?

4. Tell me in your own words what is important in this passage.

5. Look back at the paragraph. Were there any words that were new to you?

6. Look at the word *validated* in the paragraph. What kind of word is *validated*? Is it a noun, a verb, an adjective, or an adverb?

7. What does *validated* mean in this passage?

F. Whale Facts

2. What do you think this passage will be about?

The blue whale is the Earth's largest creature. Its immense body is four times larger than the biggest known dinosaur. It weighs more than 20 elephants. Unfortunately, the blue whale is in danger of becoming extinct because so many have been killed for their blubber. It is now illegal to hunt blue whales.

3. In one sentence, what is the main idea in the paragraph?

4. Tell me in your own words what is important in this passage.

5. Look back at the paragraph. Were there any words that were new to you?

6. Look at the word *immense* in the paragraph. What kind of word is *immense*? Is it a noun, a verb, an adjective, or an adverb?

7. What does *immense* mean in this passage?

G. Snowy Dangers

2. What do you think this passage will be about?

An avalanche is a very dangerous force of nature. It occurs when the pull of gravity becomes stronger than the force holding the snow onto the mountain. It usually happens after a heavy snowfall of 12 inches or more. An avalanche can travel up to 200 miles per hour and crash with tremendous force at the bottom of the mountain, causing great destruction to everything in its path.

3. In one sentence, what is the main idea in the paragraph?

4. Tell me in your own words what is important in this passage.

5. Look back at the paragraph. Were there any words that were new to you?

6. Look at the word *tremendous* in the paragraph. What kind of word is *tremendous*? Is it a noun, a verb, an adjective, or an adverb?

7. What does *tremendous* mean in this passage?

H. An Unexpected Friend

2. What do you think this passage will be about?

Bats tend to be misunderstood. They have a reputation for being dangerous and evil. In reality, bats are helpful to humans. Their diet consists of insects that are harmful to crops and which are annoying to humans. It is in our best interest to protect bats since they are so important to the environment.

3. In one sentence, what is the main idea in the paragraph?

4. Tell me in your own words what is important in this passage.

5. Look back at the paragraph. Were there any words that were new to you?

6. Look at the word *reputation* in the paragraph. What kind of word is *reputation*? Is it a noun, a verb, an adjective, or an adverb?

7. What does *reputation* mean in this passage?

I. A Cool Summer Activity

2. What do you think this passage will be about?

Inner-tubing is a popular summer activity. Rivers suitable for this are usually not very deep and have a calm flow of water. People who go "tubing" usually wear some kind of protection on their feet as well as life vests. Because of the current of the river, the inner tube does not need to be steered or rowed. The ride down the river tends to be a fun, relaxing event.

3. In one sentence, what is the main idea in the paragraph?

4. Tell me in your own words what is important in this passage.

5. Look back at the paragraph. Were there any words that were new to you?

6. Look at the word *suitable* in the paragraph. What kind of word is *suitable*? Is it a noun, a verb, an adjective, or an adverb?

7. What does *suitable* mean in this passage?

J. Biking Off-Road

2. What do you think this passage will be about?

BMX riding is a sport that has become very popular. BMX stands for bicycle motor cross. This type of bike riding is done on rugged dirt trails that have sharp turns and jumps. Competitions are held so kids can race against each other to win prizes and trophies. This sport is generally safe and provides a fun way to exercise.

3. In one sentence, what is the main idea in the paragraph?

4. Tell me in your own words what is important in this passage.

5. Look back at the paragraph. Were there any words that were new to you?

6. Look at the word *rugged* in the paragraph. What kind of word is *rugged*? Is it a noun, a verb, an adjective, or an adverb?

7. What does *rugged* mean in this passage?

Benchmark 8: The student identifies key vocabulary that helps predict the content of a passage.

Baseline 8: Read the following phrases to the student. Ask, "What does the phrase _____ tell you about what you're about to read?"

> *Note:* The targets listed for the phrases are just suggestions. Base progress on the student's ability to use context to interpret and predict the flow of the passage. Additional signal words and phrases are listed on the next page.

Phrases	*Target Responses*
for instance	It's an example.
a key feature	add to what I know
consequently	conclusion, as a result
the chief factor	It's important.
as a result	cause/effect
referred to as	definition
in contrast	the opposite from what you've read
primarily	It's important.
specifically	It's an example.
the major fact	It's important.

Here is a list of other vocabulary that signals the flow of the passage.

Add to what I know
- and
- more
- moreover
- furthermore
- besides
- some
- many
- for one thing
- likewise
- main
- another
- first
- second
- third
- also
- mainly
- primarily
- a key feature
- in addition
- next

It's Important
- better
- most
- least
- most of all
- above all
- worst
- major
- all
- few
- best
- good
- important
- chief factor
- less
- bad
- minor
- some

Comparison/Contrast
- more
- compares
- otherwise
- differences
- similar
- alike
- than
- nevertheless
- contrasts
- likeness
- similarly

Opposite
- yet
- however
- but
- otherwise
- nevertheless
- still
- in spite of
- likewise
- in contrast
- instead
- even though

Conclusion/Summary
- therefore
- thus
- finally
- in conclusion
- consequently
- hence
- as a result
- in summary
- noteworthy
- last of all

Cause/Effect
- it is because
- because
- unless
- as a result
- effect
- the quality
- attribute
- for this reason
- consequently
- if

Definition
- referred to as
- is
- the same as
- means
- termed
- defined as
- means the same
- a synonym for

Example
- for example
- to illustrate
- specifically
- for instance
- such as
- following are

> **Goal:** to improve the understanding and use of the language used in classroom material at the 7th – 12th grade levels

Benchmark 1: The student identifies the main idea of a paragraph.

Benchmark 2: The student paraphrases or summarizes a paragraph including four important details.

Benchmark 3: The student applies word recognition strategies to acquire new vocabulary and to infer meaning of an unfamiliar word.

> *Note:* If the student is reading the material independently, it should be at an appropriate reading level.

Baselines 1-3: As the student follows along, read the following paragraphs. Ask the questions (1-3) which correspond to the targeted benchmarks.

> *Note:* Although the unfamiliar words in Benchmark 3 were taken from 7th – 12th grade curriculum, they may not be unfamiliar to your student. Use your clinical judgment to determine if this skill is emerging as your student encounters novel words in text.

A. Ancient Fun

The Aztec culture played several ball games for their recreational enjoyment. One game, called Ulama, was a ball game in which the players propelled a ball from their hips, aiming the ball through rings secured to the walls of ball courts.

1. In one sentence, what is the main idea in the paragraph?

2. Tell me in your own words what is important in this passage.

3. What does *propelled* mean in this passage?

B. Early Medicine

In Colonial America it was a common belief that only one illness could affect your body at a time. This gave way to medical practices such as "blistering" in which a hot poker was placed on the skin, creating blisters. This practice was commonly performed to get rid of a cold or infection. People thought that the cold or infection would "leave" the body when the blisters were created.

1. In one sentence, what is the main idea in the paragraph?

2. Tell me in your own words what is important in this passage.

3. What does *practice* mean in this passage?

C. Copycat Houses

During the Victorian era, a popular design for homes was to imitate the Gothic style of cathedrals of the Middle Ages. Arches and spires were added to the structures of the homes which was thought to be attractive at the time. In retrospect, those designs are now regarded as hideous and unsuitable for houses.

1. In one sentence, what is the main idea in the paragraph?

2. Tell me in your own words what is important in this passage.

3. What does *hideous* mean in this passage?

D. Measuring Fitness

A treadmill test is used by physicians to determine a person's fitness level. As the patient runs on the treadmill, instruments measure how well he takes in oxygen when he breathes. As the exercise becomes more vigorous, the machine records changes in the person's ability to do harder exercise.

1. In one sentence, what is the main idea in the paragraph?

2. Tell me in your own words what is important in this passage.

3. What does *vigorous* mean in this passage?

E. A Bed of Straw

In England during the 1800s, most people slept on mattresses made of straw with a log of wood underneath as a bolster. It wasn't until around 1920 that ordinary citizens had more comfortable beds made with feather mattresses and pillows.

1. In one sentence, what is the main idea in the paragraph?

2. Tell me in your own words what is important in this passage.

3. What does *bolster* mean in this passage?

F. The Language of Dogs

Much information can be gained about a dog's disposition from his body language. If his ears are laid back and his head is down, it indicates fear or aggression. A tail between the legs shows uncertainty or submission. A dog with pert ears and an open mouth conveys being relaxed and happy. Regardless of the breed, dogs give clear signals about their moods.

1. In one sentence, what is the main idea in the paragraph?

2. Tell me in your own words what is important in this passage.

3. What does *disposition* mean in this passage?

G. Principle of Expansion

Have you ever noticed that power lines hang slackly on warm days, but they are tight on cold days? This is an example of a phenomenon called *expansion*. It occurs because the molecules in the material expand, and take up more room when heated. When large structures are built, this is taken into consideration so that buildings remain stable even when the temperature changes.

1. In one sentence, what is the main idea in the paragraph?

2. Tell me in your own words what is important in this passage.

3. What does *slackly* mean in this passage?

H. Effects of Pollution

Polluted water is a big problem across the globe. Toxic materials used in industrial processes are dumped into the Earth's rivers and oceans and are very difficult to remove. These toxins are ingested by small animals like shellfish, then by larger animals such as birds and sea lions who eat the small animals. Many efforts are underway to reduce this problem, but much progress is yet to be gained.

1. In one sentence, what is the main idea in the paragraph?

2. Tell me in your own words what is important in this passage.

3. What does *ingested* mean in this passage?

I. Disappearing Ink

During the 1100s, the monks were almost the only people who had learned to read and write. They used quill pens which needed to be refilled with ink. They generally wrote on parchment or vellum which did not preserve their writings well. It is difficult today to read documents written during that time.

1. In one sentence, what is the main idea in the paragraph?

2. Tell me in your own words what is important in this passage.

3. What does *vellum* mean in this passage?

J. The Largest Desert

The Sahara Desert is the largest desert in the world. It extends over an area as large as the United States. Its landscape is diverse with mountain ranges, rocky plateaus, valleys, and plains. People live and grow crops in the fertile areas which are known as oases.

1. In one sentence, what is the main idea in the paragraph?

2. Tell me in your own words what is important in this passage.

3. What does *fertile* mean in this passage?

Benchmark 4: The student interprets similes, metaphors, and idioms.

Baseline 4: Read the following examples of figurative language to the student. Have the student explain the meaning with or without a prompt.

Similes
1. He fell as though he had been struck by lightning.
    Prompt: How did he fall?
    Possible response: really fast/suddenly

2. She strutted like a peacock.
    Prompt: How did she walk?
    Possible response: with her back up straight, like she was proud of herself

3. His mouth was as big as an oven.
    Prompt: Tell me about his mouth.
    Possible response: really large — like he could eat a lot at one time

4. His beard covered his chest like an apron.
   Prompt: Tell me about his beard.
   Possible response: It was really wide and long, down to his stomach.

5. He turned on her like a viper.
   Prompt: How did he feel about her?
   Possible response: He suddenly got angry with her.

6. The lake was as smooth as glass.
   Prompt: Tell me about the lake.
   Possible response: There were no waves or ripples.

7. He drank so much water he felt like a balloon.
   Prompt: Tell me how he felt.
   Possible response: His stomach was stretched from drinking so much it was like it would pop. He felt full.

8. She was as nervous as a cat in a room full of rocking chairs.
   Prompt: Tell me how she was feeling/acting.
   Possible response: She was probably looking around a lot, thinking something bad was about to happen.

9. The impatient clouds hurried across the sky like ships on calm water.
   Prompt: Tell me about the clouds.
   Possible response: They were moving like they were in a hurry to get somewhere; like they were being pushed by the wind.

10. The news of his capture by the Redcoats spread like wildfire.
    Prompt: Tell me about how quickly people found out about the capture.
    Possible response: It was like one person told a lot of people, and they told many more really fast.

Metaphors
1. She is a walking encyclopedia.
   Prompt: What does this tell you about what she knows?
   Possible response: She's very smart.

2. His heart is an iceberg.
   Prompt: How does he act?
   Possible response: cold; doesn't show emotions; cruel

3. She's a magician when it comes to getting her students to do the work.
   Prompt: What does she do well?
   Possible response: It seems like magic that she gets students to work; she makes it look easy.

4. The four walls were a prison to me.
    Prompt: How did this person feel?
    Possible response: trapped, like he had no freedom

5. The words were a dagger to my heart.
    Prompt: How did the words affect this person?
    Possible response: They really hurt his feelings.

6. You are an angel for doing that.
    Prompt: What makes someone like an angel?
    Possible response: do someone a big favor; be really sweet/nice

7. You are my sunshine.
    Prompt: How would this person make you feel?
    Possible response: cheery; in a good mood; like smiling

8. The frozen lake was a skater's paradise.
    Prompt: Tell me about the lake.
    Possible response: It's all a skater could want — very smooth.

9. Her smile was a warm fire on a winter day.
    Prompt: Tell me about her smile.
    Possible response: warm and friendly; makes you feel warm and cozy

10. My life is a roller coaster.
    Prompt: Describe this person's life.
    Possible response: has some happy times and some sad times

Idioms
1. He was on pins and needles as he waited to hear his name read in the will.
    Prompt: How was he feeling?
    Possible response: very excited and hopeful that his name would be in the will, and he would inherit money

2. She kept her ear to the ground to find out the source of the new story.
    Prompt: What do you think this means about what she was doing?
    Possible response: She was paying close attention to clues about the story.

3. She seemed to be digging her own grave.
    Prompt: What was the situation for this person?
    Possible response: Her situation was getting worse, and it was her own fault.

4. They let the cat out of the bag.
    Prompt: What "got out"?
    Possible response: There was a secret that they told.

5. He was a sight for sore eyes.
   Prompt: How did the person feel who saw him?
   Possible response: glad, like she missed him, or missed seeing him

6. He put his foot in his mouth.
   Prompt: What did this person do?
   Possible response: said something he shouldn't have

7. Her blood ran cold.
   Prompt: What was her reaction?
   Possible response: scared

8. Her eyes were glued to the sidewalk.
   Prompt: How was she looking?
   Possible response: Her head was down without her eyes moving.

9. The name of the movie was on the tip of her tongue.
   Prompt: What was the problem?
   Possible response: She couldn't think of the name.

10. He'd give his right arm to go to Cancun.
    Prompt: How does this person feel about going to Cancun?
    Possible response: desperate; really wants to go, but probably won't

Benchmark 5: The student uses word mapping strategies such as "Venn diagrams" or "tree diagrams" to organize related information from the 7th – 12th grade core curriculum.

Baseline 5: Show the student one of the following outlines. Have him create a visual map showing the relationships between words. (*Note:* Not all the outlines lend themselves to both types of diagrams.)

1. Topic: *Dairy Products*

   Related words
       milk (whole, low fat, skim, acidophilus, dried milk products)
       cream (whipping cream, ice cream)
       cheese (Monterey Jack, Swiss, American, Cheddar, cream cheese)
       butter (whipped, salted)

2. Topic: *Glues*

   Types of glues
       hide: from hides of animals
               in the form of powder or small grains
               needs hot water to dissolve

bone: comes from crushed bones
         in the form of powder or small grains
         needs hot water to dissolve
fish: comes from the skins of fish
         liquid form
         loses its strength after two years

How glue is made
   cooked animal parts in water
   then filtered and concentrated

Uses of glue
   Industrial: holds furniture together
               stiffens cloth and glazes paper
               book bindings
   Domestic: crafts
               household projects

3. Topic: *Systems of Government*
   Unitary System: gives most powers to the central (national) government
                    state and local government created by central government
                    countries with unitary systems: England, France, Italy, China, and
                      Cuba
   Federal System: powers shared between the central government and state
                    governments
                    people give authority to the government
                    countries that have federal systems: U.S. , Canada, Mexico, and
                      Switzerland

4. Topic: *Schizophrenia*

Definition: severe mental disease; unpredictable disturbances in thinking

Characteristics: withdrawal from reality
                  displays no or inappropriate emotions
                  develops delusions; hears "voices"

Causes: not known for sure
                  problems in brain chemicals
                  may be hereditary

Treatment: drugs
                  psychotherapy
                  hospitalization

5. Topic: *Ways to Judge Diamonds*

    Related words
    weight: measured by the caret
    purity: absence of flaws in the diamond
    flaws: small bubbles, cracks (fissures)
    color: yellowish, blue, red, brown, green, and black
    cut: the cleaner the cut, the more valuable
    types: princess, heart, round, marquis

6. Topic: *The Body's Defense System*

    Three kinds of defenses
    Barriers
    skin: protects outer body from germs
    mucous membranes: in mouth and nose; trap germs
    tears: cover eyes; wash out debris
    stomach juices: very acidic; kill germs and disease
    bacteria: live in and on body; kill harmful germs

    Reactions
    blood vessels: give off fluid and cells that destroy bad bacteria
    fever: kills or weakens germs by raising the body's temperature

    Immune system
    white cells (including B- and T-cells)
    B- and T-cells: both recognize and attack germs
    B-cells: release antibodies that attack invader
    T-cells: protect against viruses that grow inside the body; destroy cancer cells

7. Topic: *Sources of Heat*

    Sun: most important source
                provides energy when collected on solar furnaces (creates solar energy)

    Fire: heat created when wood or fuel burns
                used to cook, provide heat; heats metals to be shaped

    Earth: heat escapes through lava from volcanoes and boiling water from geysers

    Nuclear   atomic and hydrogen bombs
    energy: produces intense heat that destroys everything around it
                not useful for producing electricity without a reactor

8. Topic: *Equipment for Horseback Riding*

Clothing
blue jeans: to protect the legs from rubbing
chaps: leather trousers that fit over jeans
boots: keep feet in stirrups
hats: for protection from wind and sun

Spurs
small wheel-like attachments worn on the heels of boots
used to give signals to the horse such as turn or run faster

Whip
used to give signals or in training
causes no pain if used correctly
Types: riding crop is like a whip, but with a large loop at the tip
hunting whip has a leather lash at the tip to control the hounds while
hunting fox

Saddle
English Saddle: padded, flatter, lighter in weight
used by professional riders
Western Saddle: wide stirrups, has a horn, more stability
used by cowhands and rodeo riders

Bridle   used to control the horse
made up of a strap and pieces that fit in the horse's mouth and pulls on the
corners of the mouth

9. Topic: *Kinds of Dancing*

Theatrical: done for onlookers
Ballet
legs and arms extend out to form designs
graceful movements to music
many movements done on the dancers' toes
Modern dance
movements in a freer form than ballet
dancers make patterns with their bodies
incorporates more personal styles

Social: done for own enjoyment
Folk dancing
part of custom and tradition of a culture
done in groups in a pattern, such as circle or line
groups often perform in costume

92

Popular dancing
    associated with a time period
    steps of dance are recorded on paper; don't differ much
    types: ballroom dancing
            court dances
            swing
            waltzes
            cha-cha

10. Topic: *Disney Entertainment*

First cartoons:
    1928: short cartoon with Mickey Mouse without sound or color
    1930: Steamboat Willie was in black and white with sound
    1931: Silly Symphonies (Mickey Mouse along with Donald Duck, Goofy, and Pluto)

Movies:
    1937: first full-length cartoon was Snow White
    1949: first "true-life" adventure was Seal Island

Theme parks:
    1955: Disneyland opened in Anaheim, CA; based on cartoon characters
    1971: Walt Disney World opened near Orlando, FL
    1982: EPCOT Center opened; featured futuristic exhibits
    1983: Disneyland opened in Tokyo, Japan
    1992: Disneyland opened in Paris, France

Benchmark 6: The student demonstrates semantic flexibility by using an expression of similar meaning to avoid repeating the same word(s) in verbal/written expression.

Baseline 6: Say to the student, "Each of these sentences or groups of sentences has a word(s) that has been repeated. Substitute another word(s) that could take the place of either of the duplicated words."

> *Note:* These sentences are not semantically wrong. The goal is to build the student's ability to use varied vocabulary in written and spoken language.

1. The *gloomy* morning was followed by a *gloomy* afternoon.

2. Her body looked *frail*, but when she carried the woman out of the burning building, they knew she was not *frail*.

3. The clamp held the piece of wood with a *firm* grasp, but it was not *firm* enough when he started sawing.

4. She gave the *reason* why she was late and her teacher accepted the *reason* as true.

5. The runners were *nervous* before the race. Their parents in the stands were even more *nervous*.

6. Frank knew he could count on his friends' *support*. They always *supported* him in his campaign.

7. The boat sailed across the *calm* lake. No one knew how long it would be *calm* before the storm brought dangerous waves.

8. The geometry scores of the two girls were *equal* and they were *equal* in algebra too. Everyone wondered who would win the math contest.

9. He had to *judge* whether the punishment was fair. He didn't know the whole story, so it was hard for him to *judge*.

10. The campers played a *joke* on the camp counselor. They had to do the dishes all week when the counselor found out they were responsible for the *joke*.

Syntax

Errors of the syntax of language have significant consequences across the spectrum of a student's education. Problems with syntax in oral language in the preliterate years become the written language deficits of the emerging writer. Without intervention, the emergent writer is then unprepared for the compositions expected at the advanced levels.

In the early grades, underdeveloped syntax skills are responsible for mistakes in noun-verb agreement, and incorrect use of plurals, possessives, and comparatives. Students with syntactical deficits consistently misunderstand directions because of complex sentence structures involving word-order sequence. As these students begin to read, comprehension typically suffers as they are confused by derivations and prefix or suffix additions to root words. Their written language is simplistic with unsupported ideas.

The benchmarks and baselines in this section provide a hierarchy of expected syntax skills for each grade level. The targets for the baselines are included in the answer key for your reference, and examples are given of acceptable answers to the more open-ended baselines. As students begin to generate written language, their productions can provide an excellent assessment tool which is generally more useful than baselines. When using written language as a measurement, you can use the baselines in this section as a supplement or as examples of a target skill.

Syntax

Kindergarten

> **Goal:** to increase the understanding and use of the structure of language in the classroom at the K grade level

Benchmark 1: The student uses noun/verb agreement correctly.

Baseline 1: Read the following sentences to the student, once with each of the choices in parentheses. Ask which word goes with the sentence.

Noun-Verb Agreement
1. The girls (is, *are*) going to school.
2. Jacob (*has*, have) been taking karate lessons.
3. The refrigerator (keep, *keeps*) food cold.
4. Robert (are, *is*) going to summer camp.
5. Her parents (walks, *walk*) with her to school.
6. Bart forgot to (*do*, does) his homework.
7. Mike (play, *plays*) soccer.
8. Ethan's mom (drive, *drives*) him to school.
9. Mrs. Best (check, *checks*) our papers.
10. Cats (*like*, likes) to lie in the sun.

Benchmark 2: The student uses singular and plural possessive pronouns correctly (e.g., *me / mine, his / her, hers, us / ours, them / theirs*).

Baseline 2: Read the following sentences aloud. Have the student supply the missing word in each sentence.

1. I gave you a book. The book is _____ (yours). The book belongs to _____ (you).
2. The bike was a gift from my dad. It is _____ (mine). It belongs to _____ (me).
3. They bought a new car. That car belongs to _____ (them). It is _____ (theirs).
4. Melissa brought her crayons to class. They are _____ (hers). They belong to _____ (her).
5. I brought Mr. Smith an apple. It is _____ (his). It belongs to _____ (him).

6. Tim and Alex won a fish at the fair. The fish is _____ (theirs). The fish belongs to _____ (them).
7. We took the chairs to the game. The chairs belong to _____ (us). They are _____ (ours).
8. Dylan gave me flowers. The flowers are _____ (mine). They belong to _____ (me).
9. Sam won the race. The trophy belongs to _____ (him). It is _____ (his).
10. The children took off their boots by the door. The boots are _____ (theirs). They belong to _____ (them).

Benchmark 3: The student uses the pronouns *he / she / they* correctly.

Baseline 3: Read the following sentences to the student. Have him answer the question following each sentence.

> *Note:* The student may need a prompt such as "Are we talking about a boy or girl? Do we know his name? What do we call him?"

1. The boy is feeding the ducks. Who is feeding the ducks? (he)

2. The girl ate her lunch. Who ate lunch? (she)

3. The kids are swinging. Who are swinging? (they)

4. The man wrote a letter. Who wrote a letter? (he)

5. The girls are flying a kite. Who are flying a kite? (they)

6. The woman is painting the fence. Who is painting the fence? (she)

7. The men sold popcorn. Who sold popcorn? (they)

8. The students are at recess. Who are at recess? (they)

9. The boys are trading cards. Who are trading cards? (they)

10. The women paid the bill. Who paid the bill? (they)

Benchmark 4: The student uses present progressives correctly.

Benchmark 5: The student uses regular past tense verbs correctly.

> **Baselines 4 and 5:** Read the following sentences to the student. Have him supply the missing words.

1. Jenn likes to skip. Now she is _____ (skipping). Yesterday Jenn _____ (skipped).

2. Chad always cleans his room. Now he is _____ (cleaning). Yesterday he _____ (cleaned).

3. Marissa loves to play with blocks. Now she is _____ (playing). Yesterday she _____ (played).

4. Carson likes to listen to music. Now he is _____ (listening). Yesterday he _____ (listened).

5. Baby Paige cries when she is hungry. She is hungry, so now she is _____ (crying). When she was hungry yesterday, she _____ (cried).

6. Luke crawls up the stairs. Now he is _____ (crawling). Yesterday he _____ (crawled).

7. Chase likes to climb trees. Now he is _____ (climbing). Yesterday he _____ (climbed).

8. Harrison likes to carry his new backpack. Now he is _____ (carrying). Yesterday he _____ (carried).

9. Kayla brushes her hair every day. Now she is _____ (brushing). Yesterday she _____ (brushed).

10. Dustin loves to cook spaghetti. Now he is _____ (cooking). Yesterday he _____ (cooked).

Goal: to increase the understanding and use of the structure of language in the classroom at the 1st grade level

Benchmark 1: The student uses contractions correctly.

Baseline 1: Have the student combine two words from each sentence to make a contraction. Provide an example if necessary.

Example: I think they are going to the movie. (they're)

Contractions
1. I am younger than my sister. (I'm)
2. She is going to the ice rink. (She's)
3. They are swimming in a race. (They're)
4. He is my only brother. (He's)
5. It is the 5th of December. (It's)
6. You should not cheat on the test. (shouldn't)
7. I could not call you yesterday. (couldn't)
8. She will not win the race. (won't)
9. I understand why you do not want to go. (don't)
10. Brent and Jill were not at the game. (weren't)

Benchmark 2: The student identifies declarative and interrogative sentences.

Baseline 2: Read the following sentences. Ask the student to say whether the sentence is declarative ("telling") or interrogative ("asking").

1. Are you going to the party? (interrogative)
2. He is a tall man. (declarative)
3. Michelle can run really fast. (declarative)
4. Why did you call your mom? (interrogative)
5. The chairs are blue. (declarative)
6. After the game, I will go home. (declarative)
7. She saw the movie yesterday. (declarative)
8. What time is it? (interrogative)
9. Where is my water bottle? (interrogative)
10. Grapes can become raisins. (declarative)

Goal: to increase the understanding and use of the structure of language in the classroom at the 2nd grade level

Benchmark 1: The student identifies nouns and verbs correctly.

    Baseline 1: Read the following list of words. Have the student identify each one as a noun or a verb.

1. cat (noun)
2. skip (verb)
3. sing (verb)
4. boy (noun)
5. Alaska (noun)
6. wear (verb)
7. closet (noun)
8. teacher (noun)
9. book (noun)
10. classroom (noun)

Benchmark 2: The student uses irregular past tense correctly.

    Baseline 2: Read the following sentences. Ask the student to fill in the missing word.

1. Today I will drink a soda. Yesterday I _____ (drank) a soda.
2. Today I will drive to the store. Yesterday I _____ (drove) to the store.
3. Today I will freeze the ice. Yesterday I _____ (froze) the ice.
4. Today I will break the record. Yesterday I _____ (broke) the record.
5. Today I will write a book. Yesterday I _____ (wrote) a book.
6. Today I will give a report. Yesterday I _____ (gave) a report.
7. Today I will speak to the teacher. Yesterday I _____ (spoke) to the teacher.
8. Today I will fly a kite. Yesterday I _____ (flew) a kite.
9. Today I will draw a picture. Yesterday I _____ (drew) a picture.
10. Today I will run the race. Yesterday I _____ (ran) the race.

Benchmark 3: The student uses irregular past tense to retell a story.

    Baseline 3: Elicit irregular past tense verbs, such as those listed below, by having the student tell the story of *Goldilocks and the Three Bears*. If he does not use five irregular verbs, probe by using the word in the infinitive form. For example, "Goldilocks went upstairs to see if there was anywhere *to sleep*. She found the beds and _____."

1. took a walk in the woods
2. went into a house
3. found porridge
4. ate the porridge
5. sat in the chairs
6. broke a chair
7. felt tired
8. slept in their beds
9. got scared when they got home
10. ran away

Goal: to increase the understanding and use of the structure of language in the classroom at the 3rd/4th grade levels

Benchmark 1: The student gives the meanings of words containing basic prefixes and suffixes (e.g., *un-, re-, dis-, pre-, uni-, bi-, tri-, trans-, -ment, -able, -ly, -ness, -ful, -er, -ist*).

> **Baseline 1:** Ask the student to determine the meanings of the words based on what he knows about prefixes and suffixes.
>
> unworthy (not worthy)   transworld (across the world)
> pretest (before the test)   disable (not able)
> distrust (fail to trust)   reorganize (organize again)
> triangle (three angles)   inaccurate (not accurate)
> misjudge (wrongly judge)   microfilm (very small film)
>
> disappointment (the "condition" of being disappointed)
> angelic ("like" an angel)
> softly (in a soft "way")
> teacher ("one who" teaches)
> doubtful ("full" of doubt)
> dirty ("full" of dirt)
> shyness (the "condition" of being shy)
> drinkable ("that can be" drunk)
> fertilize ("to make" fertile)
> friendship (the "condition" of being friends)

Benchmark 2: When presented with two sentences (one passive, one present), the student determines whether or not the sentences mean the same. If they have different meanings, the student tells how they're different.

> **Baseline 2:** Ask the student, "Do these sentences have the same or different meanings?"
>
> 1a.   The police officer arrested the thief.
> 1b.   The thief was arrested by the police officer.
>
> 2a.   The picture of Melissa was taken by Kamrie.
> 2b.   Melissa took the picture of Kamrie.
>
> 3a.   Devon read the story to Jake.
> 3b.   The story was read to Devon by Jake.

4a.   The video games were played by José.
4b.   José played video games.

5a.   Scott took out the trash.
5b.   The trash was taken out by Scott.

6a.   The team threw the pies at the coach.
6b.   The pies were thrown by the coach.

7a.   The candle was lit by the child.
7b.   The child lit the candle.

8a.   The patient was given a shot by the nurse.
8b.   The patient gave a shot.

9a.   The owner gave the puppy a bath.
9b.   The puppy was given a bath by the owner.

10a.   Tara hit the ball to Kirk.
10b.   The ball was hit to Tara.

Benchmark 3: When given a past tense sentence, the student creates a passive sentence.

Baseline 3: Instruct the student to make each sentence into a passive sentence.

1. The man carried the book bag.
2. She hit the computer keyboard.
3. Andrea picked the flowers in the yard.
4. Lauri fed the cat.
5. Maureen took her daughter to the zoo.
6. Joe paid the gas bill.
7. Karen pulled the anchor out of the water.
8. Jackie mailed the letter.
9. André mowed the lawn yesterday.
10. Tony drove the new car.

Benchmark 4: The student combines several sentences into one sentence by using complex conjoiners (e.g., *then, when, before, after, because, so if/then, but, though, although*).

Baseline 4: Say to the student, "Put the word _____ in a sentence."

then	so
when	if/then
before	but
after	though
because	although

Benchmark 5: The student uses multiple modifiers and prepositional phrases to elaborate noun phrases.

    Baseline 5: Have the student use modifiers ("describers") and prepositional phrases to add more information to the sentences.

Example: the tree
Possible new phrase: the <u>old oak</u> tree <u>next to the river</u>

1. the woman
2. a computer
3. the firefighter
4. some machines
5. a picture
6. the house
7. the camera
8. a bush
9. every duck
10. each building

Benchmark 6: The student elaborates a verb phrase by adding an adverb.

    Baseline 6: Instruct the student to expand the phrase by describing the verb.

        Note: Adverbs may be added before or after the verb.

1. Mena read _____.
2. Jeremy jumped _____.
3. The book fell _____.
4. The horse bucked _____.
5. Fish swim _____.
6. The boy cut _____.
7. She watched _____.
8. The teacher spoke _____.
9. He untied _____.
10. Pete sang _____.

Benchmark 7: The student identifies and describes sentence types according to purpose (e.g., declarative, interrogative, imperative, exclamatory).

Baseline 7: Have the student identify the following sentences by type and explain why. (Note: The end punctuation has been omitted from these sentences to avoid providing any clues.)

Example: Find the largest apple (It's an imperative sentence because someone is being told to do something.)

1. Close the closet door
2. The queen has such a big crown
3. Have you seen the latest play
4. Next week I'm going camping
5. I can't believe she won the race
6. Don't scratch the table with your fork
7. What nice shoes those are
8. Remember your brother's birthday next week
9. Which books are yours
10. The game is over

Benchmark 8: When given a topic sentence, the student adds five supporting ideas in sentence form.

Baseline 8: Have the student give five ideas that have to do with the following sentence topic.

1. Mother bears can be fierce when they believe their cubs are in danger.

Possible related ideas:
Sometimes humans try to get close to cubs.
A mother bear thinks the cubs are in danger.
She might growl, scratch with her claws, and even kill to protect her cubs.
It is best to stay away from bear cubs.
When there is a cub, there is an adult bear close by.

2. A person can learn just about anything from a book.

Possible related ideas:
Books are written on every subject.
People who know a lot about something write books.
Lots of books are written on the topics of science, geography, and history.
Books that are real or true stories are called nonfiction.
The library has many books that can be borrowed.

3. Computers have made our lives easier.

Possible related ideas:
    Computers help us do many things.
    Computers control the temperature in a house.
    Cars have computer chips to tell us when something is wrong.
    E-mail uses the computer to quickly send messages.
    Banks and stores use computers to keep track of money and sales.

4. The summer heat can be dangerous to pets.

Possible related ideas:
    Pets with fur don't sweat like humans.
    If pets don't drink enough water, they could die from thirst.
    The sun can cause heat stroke or dehydration.
    Pets should never be left in a hot car.
    Many pets die each year from too much heat.

5. Recycling is an easy way to care for the environment.

Possible related ideas:
    When we recycle we use things again instead of throwing them away.
    Plastic, aluminum, glass, and paper can be recycled.
    People take their recyclable items to recycle centers to get money.
    Some communities have curbside recycling.
    The more we can reuse our environment, the less we waste.

6. School is a great place to make friends.

Possible related ideas:
    Kids in the same grade are all about the same age.
    Kids the same age like to do many of the same things.
    If you have a friend in your class, you can do projects together.
    There are a lot of things to do on the playground with friends like jumping rope,
      playing tetherball, and climbing bars.
    School is a place where you can make a friend for life.

7. Bread is shaped in many different ways.

Possible related ideas:
    Before bread is baked, the dough is easy to shape.
    Bread can be shaped like a stick, called a breadstick, or into a round loaf.
    Bread can be braided like challah or folded like a croissant.
    Rolls are small breads and can be round, square, or stacked like Zwieback.
    Whatever the shape, bread is best when it's fresh from the oven.

8. Following the playground rules is important.

Possible related ideas:
    The rules on the playground help keep everyone safe.
    If someone breaks a rule, someone might get hurt.
    For example, climbing up the slide is dangerous if someone is sliding down.
    Some kids think the rules keep them from having fun.
    It is more fun to play when no one gets hurt.

9. Jungle animals are very different from farm animals.

Possible related ideas:
    Jungle animals' bodies help them reach food because they have to get it themselves.
    For example, the giraffe has a long neck and a long tongue to reach leaves in the trees.
    The colors of jungle animals help them blend into the background and keep them safe.
    Many jungle animals move faster than farm animals.
    The cheetah runs fast to catch its food, and the gazelle runs fast to get away from the cheetah.

10. There are many ways to travel across the country.

Possible related ideas:
    The bus and car travel on roads.
    Trains travel on tracks.
    Airplanes are the fastest way to travel.
    Airline tickets cost the most, but then you get where you are going faster.
    Most people choose how they want to travel based on time and money.

Goal: to increase the understanding and use of the structure of language in the classroom at the 5th/6th grade levels

Benchmark 1: The student identifies propositions included in a complex sentence taken from classroom context or newspaper stories.

Baseline 1: Have the student identify the separate ideas in the complex sentences.

Note: The order and structure of the propositions given aren't the only possibilities. Judge the benchmark as met if the student is able to identify all of the ideas in the sentence.

1. A 4-week-old opossum, whose mother was killed by a car, feeds from a tiny bottle at the California Wildlife Center.

2. Detroit school officials will replace much of a $2 million air-conditioning system at Washington High School because of complaints from parents.

3. California is one of only 12 states where theme parks aren't subject to state inspections or required to open their accident records.

4. The Lexington Library will announce today that it has acquired the complete writings of the British-born author Felix Hebert.

5. As video game sales continue to skyrocket, analysts predict that for the first time ever people will spend more on electronic entertainment this year than at movie theaters.

6. Rebuilding the city's number one attraction seems to be easier than finding the cause for the huge November fire that destroyed a quarter of the Wharf.

7. Other passengers, mostly women in their 70s and 80s, suffered either serious or minor injuries in the wreck.

8. Details of the robbery case, now in the hands of a San Antonio grand jury, were reported by Dallas Daily News.

9. Spears College's baseball team will open the six-team playoffs against Charter University in Caldwill, Idaho.

10. Deputies from the Sheriff's Office are investigating a hit-and-run accident that occurred when the driver of a vehicle ran into a parked car.

Benchmark 2: Given several phrases, the student creates complex sentences.

> **Baseline 2:** Have the student arrange the phrases in a logical order to construct complex sentences.

> > *Note:* To help the student judge whether or not the sentence makes sense, write each phrase of the complex sentence on a separate card and have the student move them around.

1. when she heard who the judges would be
   she became even more nervous
   about trying out for the school play

2. during the winter
   in New Jersey
   it's hard to drive in the snow
   without 4-wheel drive

3. with several servings of fruit a day
   health experts say
   which you can easily get from the grocery store
   you can improve your general health

4. without reading a newspaper
   you can get the daily news
   if you listen to the radio
   which airs the top stories

5. in the mall
   at the edge of town
   I bought a new sweater
   off the sale rack

6. we still couldn't get out the stain
   that was left by the red punch
   even after scrubbing the rug
   at the party

7. on Friday afternoons
   at Mountainview Elementary
   Del's lemonade is sold
   to thirsty children

8. it is important to use the crosswalk
   when crossing a busy street
   because it is the safest way to cross
   and it's against the law to jaywalk

9. after presenting the awards
   the coach thanked the parents
   because of their dedication to the team
   at last night's banquet

10. because the class sounded interesting
    I decided to enroll
    in the line-dancing class
    at the College of the Canyons

Benchmark 3: The student expands sentence length by adding relative clauses (e.g., *where, who, that, which, when*) to noun phrases.

Baseline 3: Have the student add a clause that adds information to the noun phrase.

Note: If needed as a cue, a "starter" is provided in parentheses.

Example: Bill's shoes were missing.
Bill's shoes, which he usually kept by the door, were missing.

1. Mr. Jenkins, *(who _____)*, is a popular teacher.
2. The seagull, *(that _____)*, flew away with my sandwich.
3. The 4th of July, *(when _____)*, is celebrated with fireworks.
4. Washington D.C., *(where _____)*, has cold winters.
5. Chocolate cake, *(which _____)*, was served for his birthday.
6. The river, *(that _____)*, flooded last spring.
7. The artist, *(who _____)*, opened a new art gallery.
8. Clean water, *(which _____)*, is important for good health.
9. Wednesday evenings, *(when _____)*, I do the dishes.
10. Hart Park, *(where _____)*, has five baseball fields.

> **Goal:** to increase the understanding and use of the structure of language in the classroom at the 7th – 12th grade levels

Benchmark 1: The student combines several related sentences from a story or article using complex conjunctions.

> *Note:* The following list of complex conjunctions is based on a hierarchy of difficulty.
>
> temporal relations with conjunctions (*then, when, before, after, while*)
> causal relations with conjunctions (*because, so*)
> conditional relations with conjunctions (*if/then*)
> notice-perception relations with "wh" conjunctions (*who, when, where*)
> specification relations with conjunctions (*that, which*)
> adversative relations with conjunctions (*but, though, although*)

Baseline 1: Have the student combine the ideas (propositions) of two sentences with the given complex conjunctions.

> *Note:* Some of the words in the original two sentences may not need to be used in the new sentence. For some items, there may be more than one correct answer.

Temporal clauses: (*while, then, when, before, after*)

1. Six years ago, the Cougars won their first championship.
   At that time, their team was undefeated.

Example: Six years ago, *when* their team was undefeated, the Cougars won their first championship.

2. The country was under communist rule.
   The War of 1887 ended communism.

3. The citizens marched outside the building.
   The mayor met with city officials at the same time.

4. Catherine the Great was a Russian ruler.
   Russia had great success immediately after she came to power.

5. He spent five years in Vermont as a child.
   He moved to New Hampshire in his teenage years.

Causal clauses: (*because, so*)

1. Melissa had a hard time seeing the board.
   Her mother took her to the eye doctor.

Example: *Because* Melissa had a hard time seeing the board, her mother took her to the
   eye doctor.

2. The air had a strange smell.
   The students reported the smell to their teacher.

3. Some people who run like to watch TV while they exercise.
   Fitness clubs have placed TV sets above the treadmill equipment.

4. He didn't have enough money with him to pay for lunch.
   He borrowed from a friend.

5. The book had a stain on the cover.
   She asked the clerk to give her a discount on the price.

Conditional clauses: (*if/then*)

> *Note:* Although *if/then* is the target relationship, the word *then* may
> not be necessary to understand the relationship.

1. The baseball game goes longer than expected.
   Jamie will miss her bus ride back to school.

Example: *If* the baseball game goes longer than expected, Jamie will miss her bus ride
   back to school.

2. Ballet becomes popular with more teenagers.
   Dance schools will have to increase the number of instructors.

3. More people may carpool.
   Gas continues to get more expensive.

4. The measure would have been passed.
   More Americans knew about the issue.

5. There is a positive review of the film.
   It will be shown as part of a class assignment.

Notice-perception clauses: (*who, when, where*)

1. Florence Nightingale was a nurse in the Crimean War.
   Soldiers called her "the lady with the lamp."

Example: Florence Nightingale, *who* was a nurse in the Crimean War, was called "the lady with the lamp" by the soldiers.

2. 1948 remains an important date in Israel's history.
   In 1948 Israel became a nation.

3. New Zealand held the largest teddy bear picnic in 1994.
   Outdoor activities are popular in New Zealand.

4. The soil in the coastal region is fertile.
   Vegetation in the coastal region is plentiful.

5. The famous baseball player gave a press conference.
   He just beat the world's record for the fastest pitch.

Specification clauses: (*that, which*)

1. Air mail was delivered by army pilots.
   Air mail required an extra charge.

Example: Air mail *that* was delivered by army pilots required an extra charge.

2. The popular television show starred Martha Long.
   The show lasted until 1978.

3. The MVP award was given to Reggie Simmons.
   The award is the most popular.

4. The dance called the waltz was outlawed in some places at first.
   It was first danced in England.

5. The Central Union Pacific Railroad was the first to extend from coast to coast.
   It was finished in 1869.

Adversative clauses: (*even though, but, although*)

1. The high school team finished in last place last season.
   The coach made winning a championship a top priority this season.

Example: *Although* the high school team finished in last place last season, the coach made winning a championship a top priority this season.

2. His father took him to see the movie last year.
   He forgot the main characters.

3. The concert was for a good cause.
   The concert still was expensive.

4. The store had a clearance sale on jackets.
   It only lasted three hours.

5. The new mayor seemed to be popular.
   She only won the election by 50 votes.

Benchmark 2: The student produces written language* with an average T-unit of 10, 11, or 12 using core curricular materials.

Grade Level	T-unit Target
8	10
10	11
12	13

Baseline 2: Obtain a written sample* (e.g., journal entry, creative writing sample, book report, written narrative) from the student. Analyze the written work sample. To figure the T-unit:

1. Divide the sample into clauses which can "stand on their own."
2. Count the words in each clause.
3. Divide by the number of clauses counted.

Example 1:
Mary and Joan went to the store and bought eggs.

1. This sentence cannot be divided into clauses.
2. There is 1 clause with 10 words.
3. 10 divided by 1 is 10. The T-unit for this sentence is 10.

* Written language may be that which the student himself wrote, or which was dictated. If visual processing problems co-exist with language problems, a dictated sample may be a better measure of the student's use of syntax.

For a complete description of the T-unit measurement, refer to:
   Lund D. and J. Duchan. *Assessing Children's Language in Naturalistic Contexts*. Englewood Cliffs, NJ: Prentice-Hall, 1993.

Example 2:
Mary and Joan went to the store (and) they bought eggs.

1. This sentence can be divided into two clauses (joined by the word *and*).
2. There are 2 clauses with 10 words. (You don't count the conjunction *and* that joins the clauses.)
3. 10 divided by 2 is 5. The T-unit for this sentence is 5.

Benchmark 3: The student recognizes root words and creates a derivative from a root word.

Baseline 3: Ask the student, "What is the root (or main) word in _____? Can you think of any other words that sound the same or have the same root word as _____?"

Word	Root	Derivatives
dramatic	drama	drama, dramatical
analyst	analyze	analysis
expensive	expense	expend, inexpensive
competitors	compete	competition
resigned	resign	resignation
valuable	value	invaluable
decision	decide	decisive, indecision
mistaken	mistake	mistakable, unmistakable
judicial	judge	judgment
limited	limit	unlimited, limitless

Voice

Clear voice production contributes to academic success in the listening and speaking curricular areas. When a student is able to convey her ideas and emotions without the interference of poor voice quality, she is a better communicator. Chronic hoarseness hinders a student's verbal effectiveness in class discussion as well as peer interaction. Poor voice quality draws attention to speech production (i.e., how the student is speaking) rather than the verbal message (i.e., what the student is saying).

The benchmarks and baselines in this unit focus on remediating the hyper-function of the vocal mechanism generally caused by vocal abuse in the school-aged child. As with other areas of speech intervention, improvement in the quality of voice is dependent on the level of the student's motivation. Several of the benchmarks leading to the goal of increasing communicative effectiveness focus on educating the student about the physiology of the voice and the effects of vocal abuse. This serves to help the student realize her contribution to therapy and hopefully increase motivation. Likewise, a benchmark for keeping a log of vocal behaviors holds the student accountable for behavior changes. The other benchmarks focus on relaxation and using "easy voicing" techniques in a hierarchy of tasks. Of course, a medical assessment to determine prognosis of intervention is an important part of voice treatment.

Voice

> **Goal:** to improve communicative effectiveness by decreasing vocal hoarseness and vocal abuse

Education

Benchmark 1: The student describes the anatomy and physiology of the larynx, vocal cords, and diaphragm when questioned by the clinician.

    Baseline 1: Have the student describe how speech is produced.

    Target: A muscle under the lungs helps you fill your lungs with air. The air comes up from the lungs, vibrates through the vocal cords in the larynx (making sound), and comes through the mouth or nose. Then the sound is shaped by the tongue, lips, and shape of the mouth.

Benchmark 2: The student describes the condition of abused vocal folds when questioned by the clinician.

    Baseline 2: Have the student describe damaged vocal cords.

    Example: "Tell me what hurt vocal cords/folds are like."

    Target: red, swollen, blistered, have bumps, feel sore, raw

Benchmark 3: The student identifies problems due to a damaged voice when questioned by the clinician.

    Baseline 3: Have the student explain problems he has pinpointed that are the result of a hoarse voice.

    Example: "What kinds of problems do you have when you've been harmful to your voice?"

    Target: My throat feels sore or dry; my voice sounds bad; people can't understand me very well; they listen to how my voice sounds instead of what I have to say.

Benchmark 4: The student demonstrates deep diaphragmatic breathing when instructed by the clinician.

    Baseline 4: Instruct the student to demonstrate the breathing techniques discussed in therapy.

    Example: "Show me the best way of getting air for talking."

    Target: breathing with movement in the abdominal area, straight torso, no movement in chest, etc.

Benchmark 5: The student demonstrates and explains the benefits of relaxation of the face, neck, and shoulder muscles when questioned by the clinician.

    Baseline 5: Instruct the student to show the relaxation techniques targeted in therapy and to talk about their benefits.

    Example 1: "Show me the way you've practiced relaxing parts of your body."

    Target: demonstration of relaxation techniques

    Example 2: "Why is relaxation important?"

    Target: When I feel stress/pressure my body gets tight and my voice gets tight too. If I can relax my muscles, my voice will get better.

Benchmark 6: The student identifies vocally abusive behaviors for _____ (period of time) using a log with the help of parent/teacher and reports behaviors to the clinician.

    Baseline 6: Have the student track daily activities when vocally abusive behaviors occur using a journal or log. Then at the end of the specified time, have the student turn in the log.

    Example: "What kinds of things do you do that are harmful to your voice?"

    Target: I imitate car noises, scream on the playground, talk too loud, etc.

Benchmark 7: The student describes alternates to each identified vocally abusive behavior when questioned by the clinician.

    Baseline 7: Have the student describe behaviors to replace those identified as vocally abusive.

        Example: "What are some good things you can do for your voice instead of those that harm your voice?"

        Target: walk over to people instead of yell at them, clap or whistle at games instead of screaming, etc.

Benchmark 8: The student describes good vocal hygiene habits when questioned by the clinician.

    Baseline 8: Question the student about vocal hygiene habits discussed in therapy.

    Example: "What can you do every day to keep your voice healthy?"

    Target: drink plenty of water during the day, stay away from smoke, use alternate behaviors for yelling, etc.

Benchmark 1: The student keeps a log of good vocal hygiene on a daily basis for _____ (designated period of time), demonstrating use of good vocal hygiene.

   Baseline 1: The student's daily log shows evidence of daily use of habits (e.g., drank glass of water, went outside when my dad started to smoke, etc.).

Benchmark 2: The student reduces laryngeal and vocal tract tension using phonation on a "sigh" or "yawn-sigh" when instructed by the clinician.

   Baseline 2: Instruct the student to demonstrate this technique.

      Example: "Show me how you can loosen up your throat when it feels tight."

      Target: phonation (e.g., "ah") with a sigh or yawn-sigh

Benchmark 3: The student uses "easy" ("light/smooth") voice production while coordinating airflow and phonation with 90% accuracy in:

   A. "h" words
   B. "h" words without the "h"
   C. "h" sentences
   D. sentences
   E. structured activities
   F. spontaneous conversation

   Baseline 3 (A, B, C): Have the student read or repeat the following words and sentences.

      Note: You may want to tape record the student to compare vocal quality production from task to task.

   A. "h" words

handy	hat	harm	heat	heel
has	high	his	heart	hit

   B. "h" words minus the "h"

Andy	at	arm	eat	eel
as	I	is	art	it

C. "h" sentences

Her favorite hat is heather-blue.
My head hurt after I bumped it.
The hound howled at the moon.
Helen scraped her heel.
He pulled the alarm in the hall.

Heath hid the handkerchief.
He jumped the high hurdle.
Heaps of hair were stuck in the sink.
He held her hand.
The heater was hot.

Baseline 3D: Have the student use "easy" ("light/smooth") voice production in sentences. For example, have the student make up a sentence about a picture or create a sentence when given a word.

Baseline 3E: Listen for easy voice production during structured activities (picture description, storytelling, reading aloud, greetings, etc. taken from core curricular material).

Baseline 3F: Listen for easy voice production (and little or no hoarseness) in spontaneous conversation.

Voice

The SLP's IDEA Companion   120

Word-Finding

The academic environment demands cohesive, quick responses. When a student is called upon in class he only has seconds to clearly state an answer or make his point in an argument. In the early years of grade school, the "wait-time" is much longer than in the upper grades, and much scaffolding is provided to help the student express himself. As a student goes through school, the wait-time allowed by teachers and peers decreases, and the responsibility of verbal communication is placed more heavily on the student. Furthermore, the importance of expressing oneself in a succinct manner occurs in many contexts (e.g., when participating in debates, in verbal banter with peers, giving the punch line to a joke).

In class discussions, if a student hesitates or fumbles the intended words, he may be "passed over" in order for another student to state the answer more clearly. If a student is unsure or frustrated because he doesn't know the answer, he may simply mumble, "I forgot." Because of the ramifications of retrieval problems, word-finding is an important area of intervention.

The benchmarks and baselines in this unit are retrieval tasks drawn from common word-finding strategies. The subjects and vocabulary used are at the third grade level so the tasks are appropriate for students functioning at or above this level. When working with younger students, adapt the vocabulary and subject matter to insure that you're measuring word-finding and not semantics.

Word-Finding

Goal: to increase the recall of known vocabulary to improve the expression of ideas in the classroom

Benchmark 1A: The student fills in a semantically-appropriate word in a cloze sentence.

Benchmark 1B: The student provides several semantically-similar words given a word in context.

Benchmark 2: The student increases the number of responses provided over trials during a timed exercise.

Baselines 1A and 1B: Read the prompt to the student. Have her provide a word that makes sense, and then give several more words that would also fit. Some possibilities are listed below each cloze sentence.

Baseline 2: Ask the student to provide as many words that fit as possible in a specific time period (e.g., 5 seconds).

1. When I go to the beach, I pack my _____.
   sunscreen   swimsuit   towel   sunglasses

2. I forgot to put _____ in the washing machine.
   laundry soap   bleach   fabric softener   clothes

3. He was going to send his friend a letter, but he didn't have _____.
   an envelope   the address   a stamp   paper   a pen/pencil

4. Jesse wanted to build a campfire, but he couldn't find _____.
   wood   a match   a fire pit   paper

5. I really like _____ on my hamburger.
   cheese   tomatoes   onions   pickles   lettuce

6. After I wake up, I always _____.
   eat breakfast   get dressed   take a shower   make my bed

7. When she made her sandwich, she put _____ on the bread.
   mayonnaise   mustard   peanut butter   jam   meat

8. She made a picture for her grandma using _____.
   paints   markers   pencils   crayons   chalk

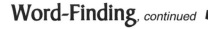

9. I was going to set the table, but I didn't know where my aunt kept her _____.
   silverware   dishes   glasses   tablecloth   napkins

10. She was looking for the keys to the _____.
    car   truck   van   door   house

Benchmark 3: The student predicts a word based on phonological properties such as syllable count (3A), rhyme (3B), or initial phoneme cue (3C).

   Baselines 3A, 3B, and 3C: Follow the prompts corresponding with syllable count, rhyme, or initial phoneme.

   Baseline 3A: Syllable Count

   1. Name something that is green and that has one syllable. (grapes, grass, tree, plants)
   2. Name a pet that has two syllables. (puppy, kitten, hamster, rabbit, turtle, goldfish)
   3. Name a cereal that has three syllables. (*Note:* the cereal name may contain more than one word.) (Cheerios, Captain Crunch, Lucky Charms, Rice Krispies)
   4. Name something on a bed that has two syllables. (pillow, blanket, covers, bedspread)
   5. Name a planet that has three syllables. (Mercury, Uranus, Jupiter)
   6. Name something that gives light that has one syllable. (lamp, fire, sun, spark)
   7. Name something you plug in that has three syllables. (radio, microwave, telephone, computer)
   8. Name something you wear that has one syllable. (shirt, pants, hat, coat, shoes)
   9. Name something you write with that has two syllables. (pencil, crayon, marker)
   10. Name a fruit that has one syllable. (peach, plum, grape, orange)

   Baseline 3B: Rhyme

   1. Name a part of a bike that rhymes with *medal*. (pedal)
   2. Name a taste that rhymes with *power*. (sour)
   3. Name a sport that rhymes with *locker*. (soccer)
   4. Name the season that rhymes with *plumber*. (summer)
   5. Name something you drink out of that rhymes with *slug*. (mug)
   6. Name something you sit on that rhymes with *wrench*. (bench)
   7. Name a part of your face that rhymes with *leak*. (cheek)
   8. Name a zoo animal that rhymes with *wheel*. (seal)
   9. Name a piece of jewelry that rhymes with *string*. (ring)
   10. Name a bird that rhymes with *love*. (dove)

   Baseline 3C: Initial Phoneme

   1. Name a fruit that starts with /s/. (strawberry)
   2. Name something you drink that starts with /w/. (water)
   3. Name something you ride on that starts with /b/. (bike)

4. Name something that has to do with weather that starts with /r/. (rain)
5. Name the part of a flower that starts with /p/. (petal)
6. Name a color that starts with /g/. (green, gold)
7. Name something that is round that starts with /w/. (wheel)
8. Name a flower that starts with /r/. (rose)
9. Name something in your desk that starts with /p/. (pencil)
10. Name a part of a shoe that starts with /l/. (lace)

Benchmark 4: The student improves word recall by naming more items of a category over trials.

Baseline 4: Instruct the student to name all the items she can think of in the listed category. Allow ten seconds. Record the number of items recalled, and compare to future baselines. Judge the benchmark as met if the student recalls more items over trials.

1. things you would find at school
2. vegetables
3. furniture
4. farm animals
5. kinds of shoes
6. sports
7. family members
8. things found in the ocean
9. weather words
10. brands of soda pop

Benchmark 5: The student reduces the time needed to name places and occupations associated with actions over trials.

Baseline 5: Set a timer. Have the student name the places or occupations associated with five of the following items. Judge the benchmark as met if the time required to complete the task is less than the original baseline.

1. This is who puts out a fire. (firefighter)
2. This is who writes a book. (author)
3. This is someone who works at a hospital. (doctor, nurse, x-ray technician)
4. This is where a dog might sleep. (doghouse, bed)
5. This is where you go to check out a book. (library)
6. This is where you go to send a letter. (post office)
7. This is where baseball is played. (baseball field, stadium)
8. This is where you go to buy plants. (nursery, store)
9. This is who takes pictures for a living. (photographer)
10. This is who you give your money to when you buy something in a store. (clerk, salesperson)

Picture Stories

Look at these pictures. They tell a story. Cut the pictures apart. Then put them back in order and tell the story.

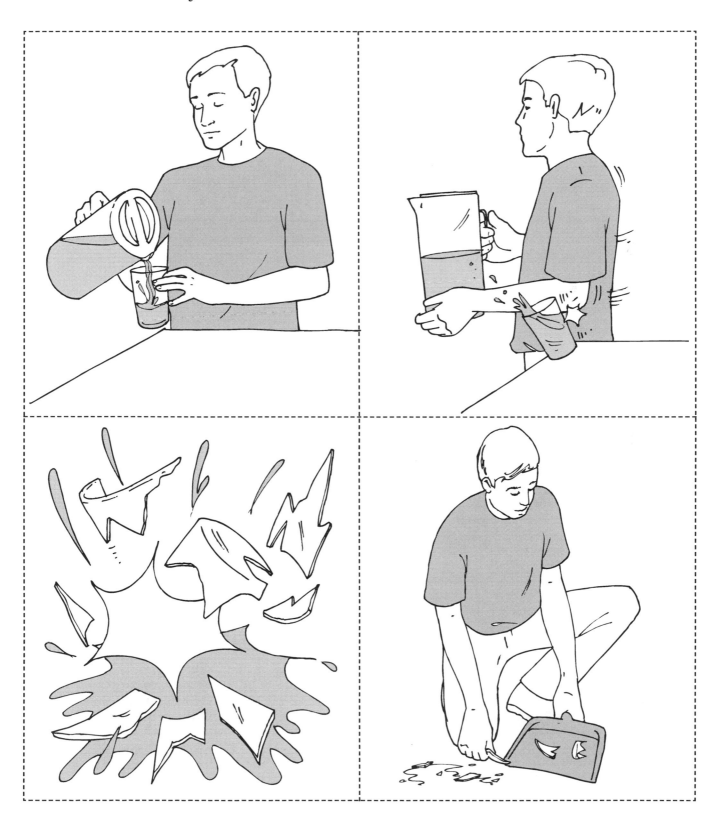

Look at these pictures. They tell a story. Cut the pictures apart. Then put them back in order and tell the story.

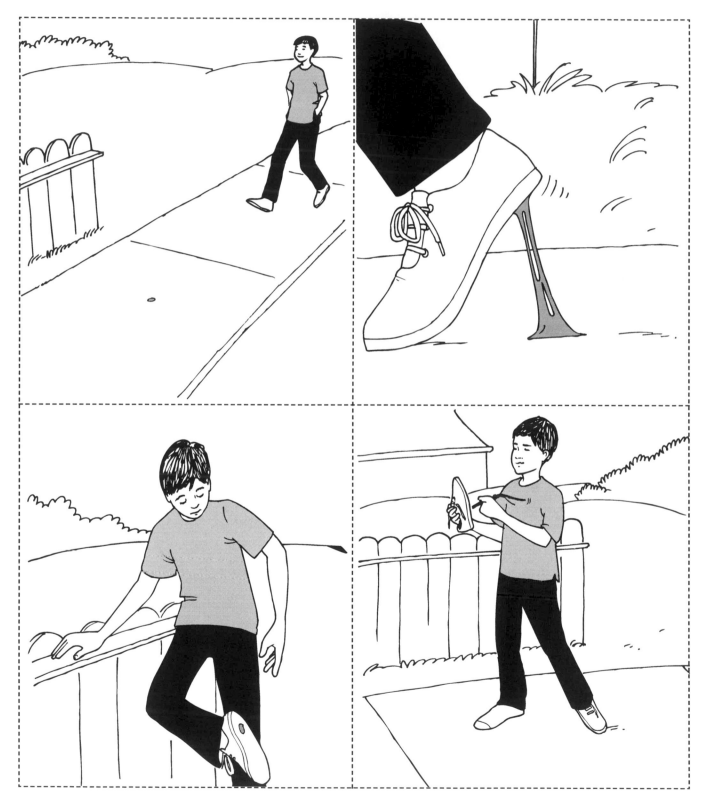

Look at these pictures. They tell a story. Cut the pictures apart. Then put them back in order and tell the story.

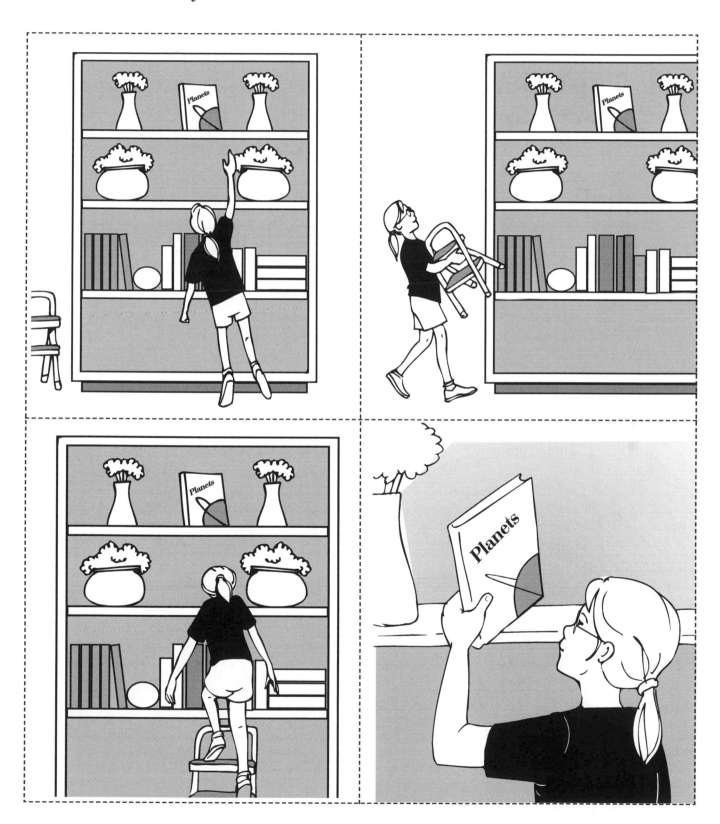

Look at these pictures. They tell a story. Cut the pictures apart. Then put them back in order and tell the story.

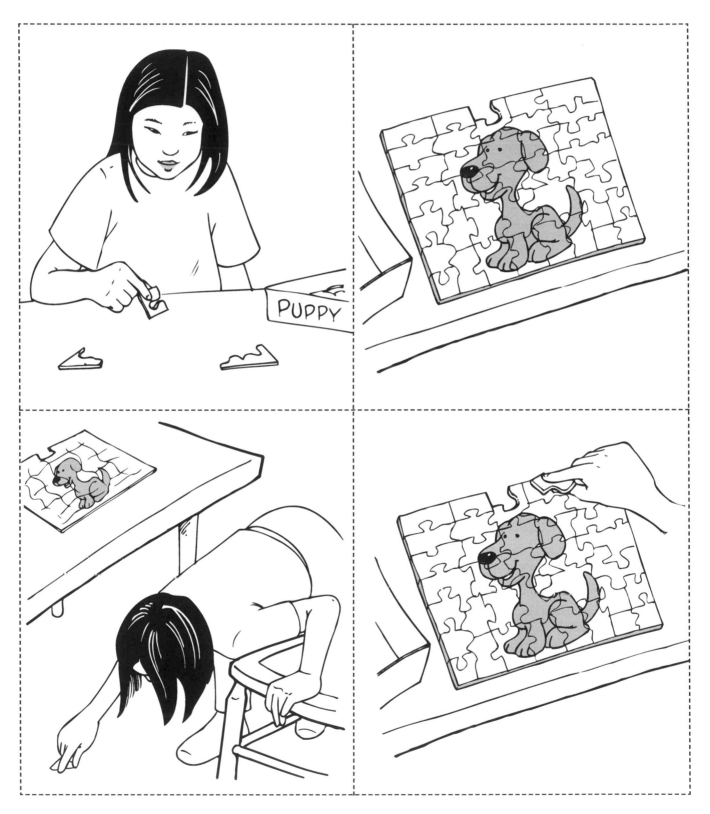

128

Look at these pictures. They tell a story. Cut the pictures apart. Then put them back in order and tell the story.

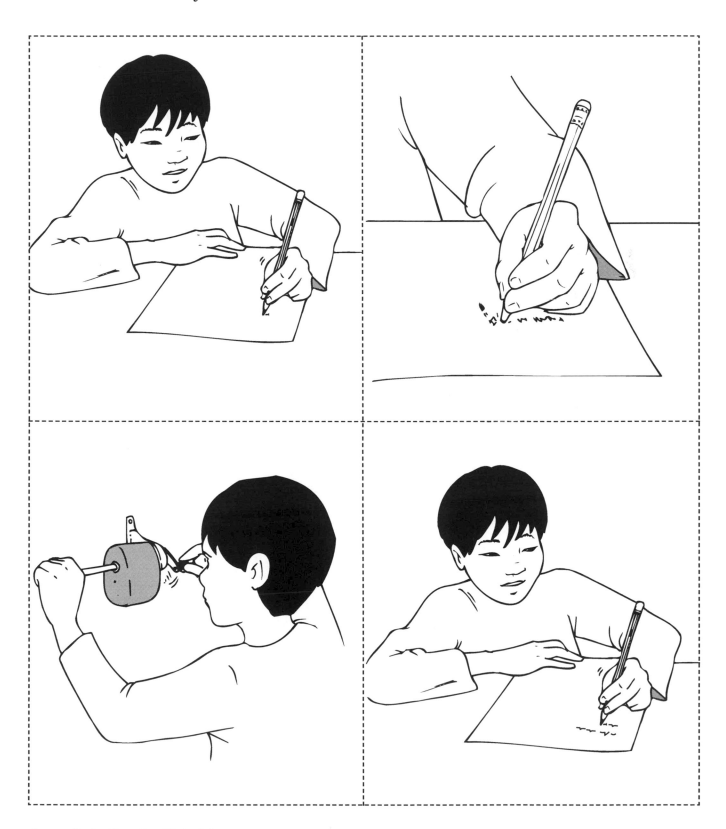

129

Look at these pictures. They tell a story. Cut the pictures apart. Then put them back in order and tell the story.

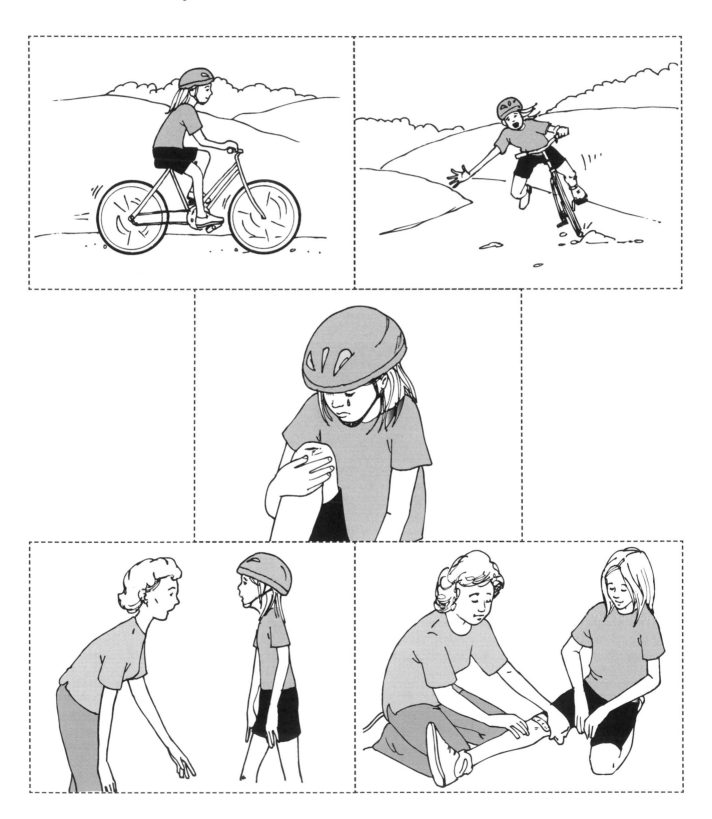

130

Look at these pictures. They tell a story. Cut the pictures apart. Then put them back in order and tell the story.

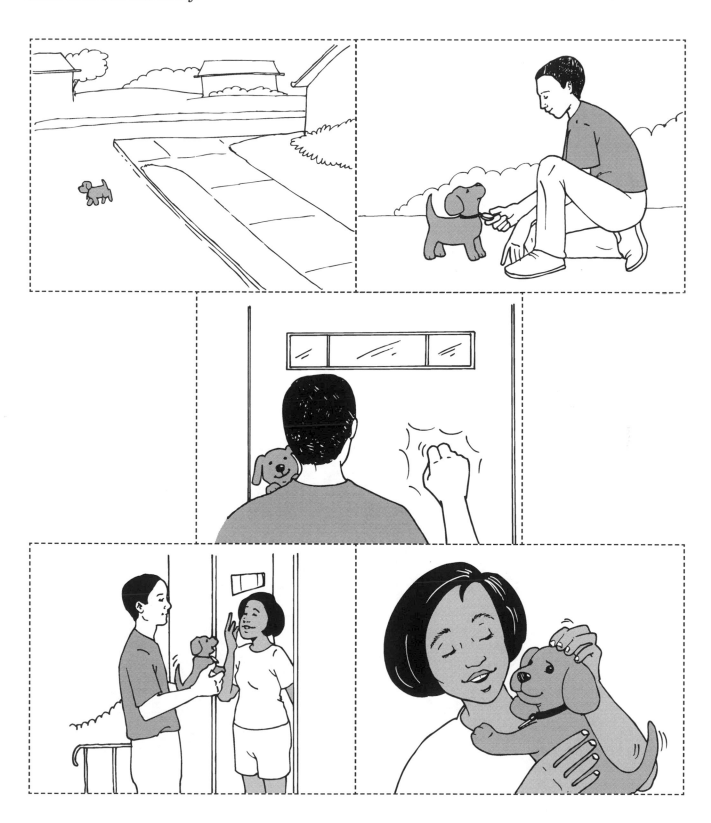

Look at these pictures. They tell a story. Cut the pictures apart. Then put them back in order and tell the story.

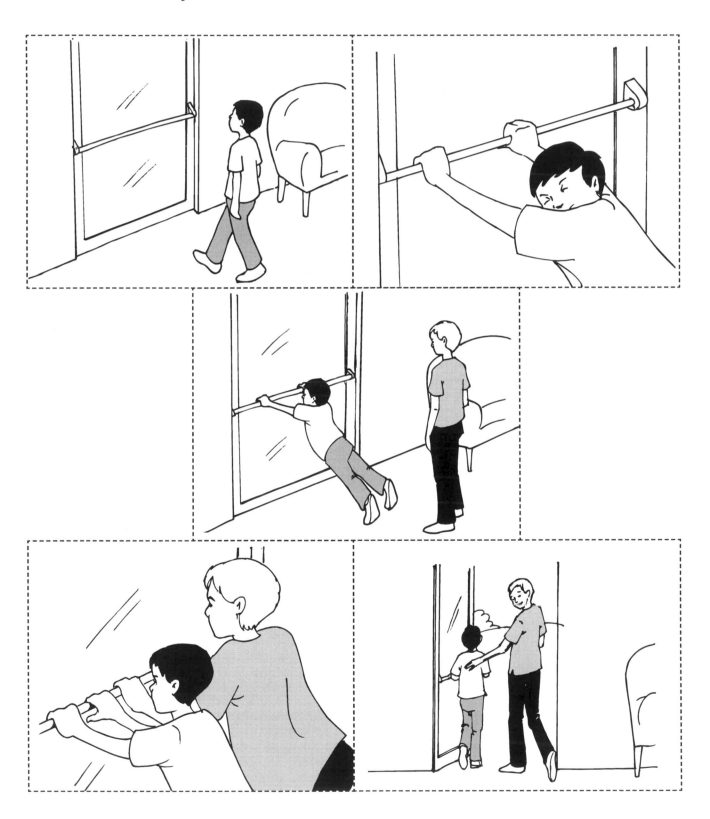

Look at these pictures. They tell a story. Cut the pictures apart. Then put them back in order and tell the story.

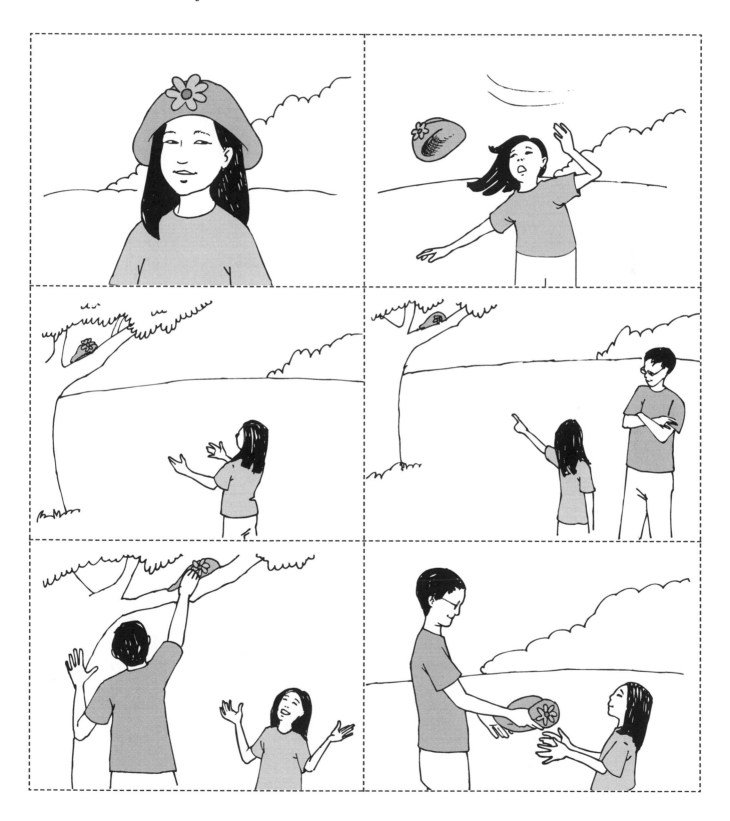

Look at these pictures. They tell a story. Cut the pictures apart. Then put them back in order and tell the story.

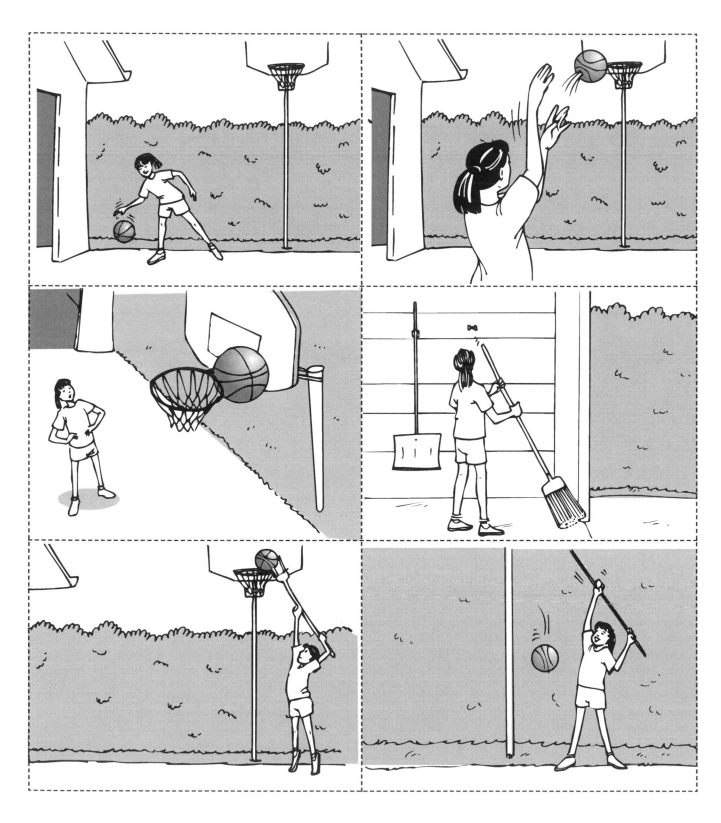

Category Pictures

Look at the pictures in each box. Find the picture that doesn't belong with the others. Then tell why it doesn't belong.

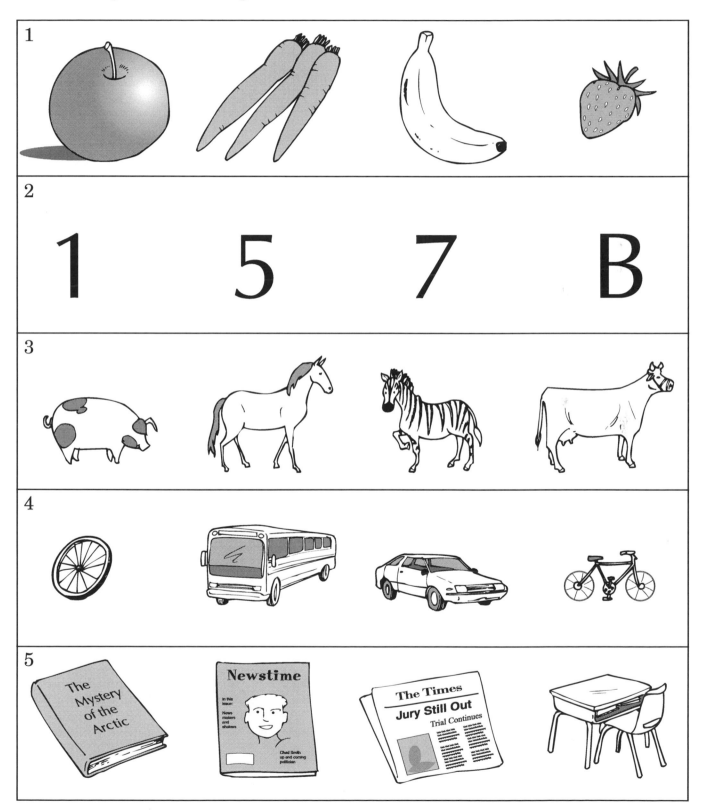

1

2

1   5   7   B

3

4

5

The Mystery of the Arctic

Newstime
In this issue:
News makers and shakers
Chad Smith up and coming politician

The Times
JURY STILL OUT
Trial Continues

Look at the pictures in each box. Find the picture that doesn't belong with the others.
Then tell why it doesn't belong.

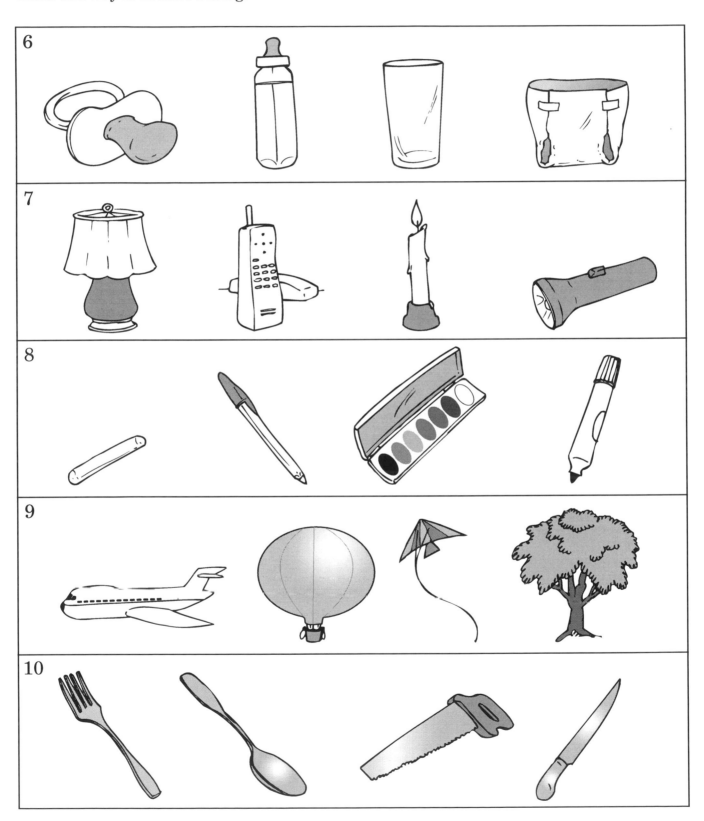

Problem Pictures

Look at these pictures. What is the problem in each picture? Why do you think it happened?

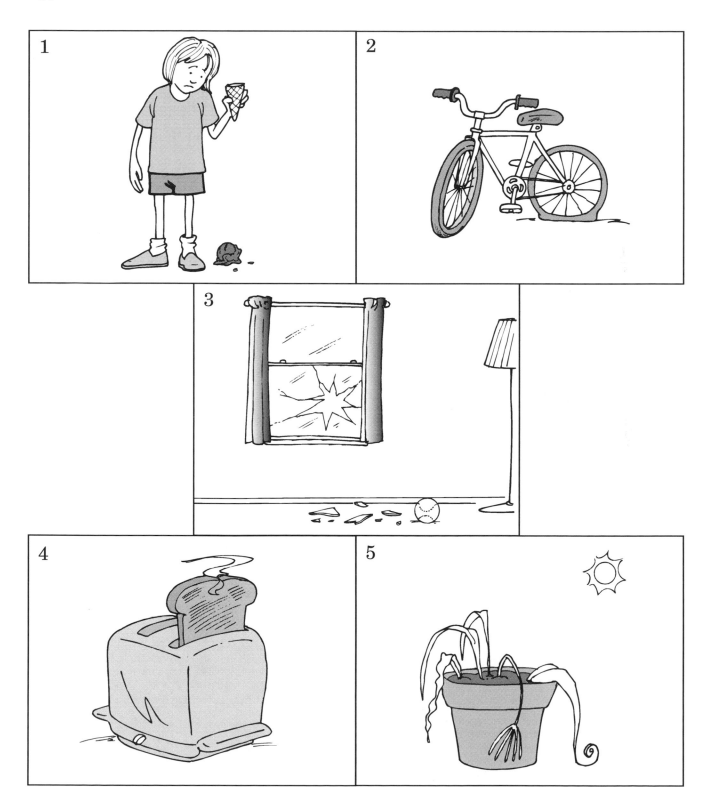

Look at these pictures. What is the problem in each picture? Why do you think it happened?

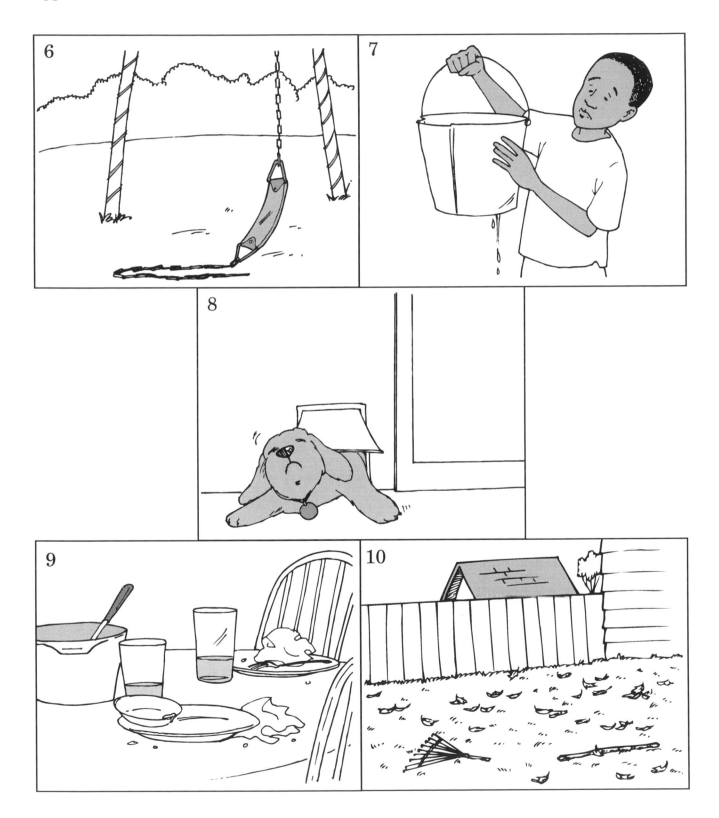

What If Pictures

Look at these pictures. What do you think might happen next?

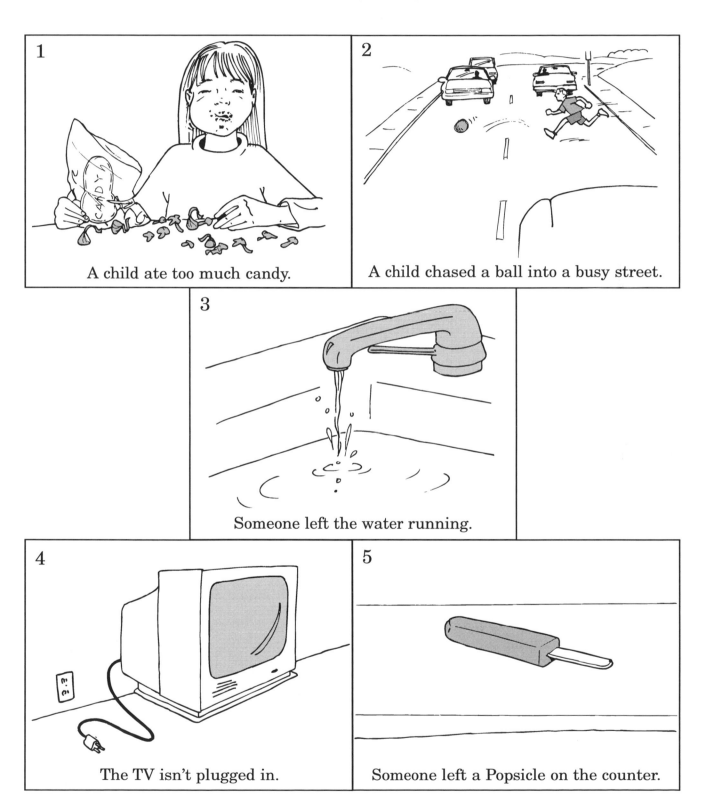

1. A child ate too much candy.

2. A child chased a ball into a busy street.

3. Someone left the water running.

4. The TV isn't plugged in.

5. Someone left a Popsicle on the counter.

Look at these pictures. What do you think might happen next?

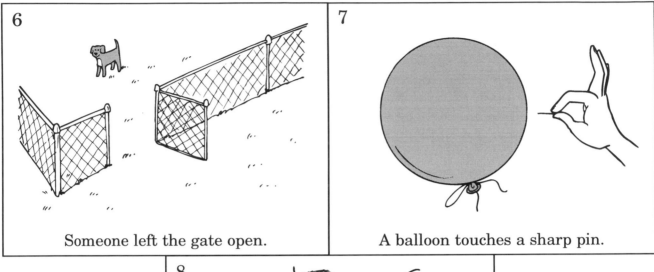

6	7
Someone left the gate open.	A balloon touches a sharp pin.

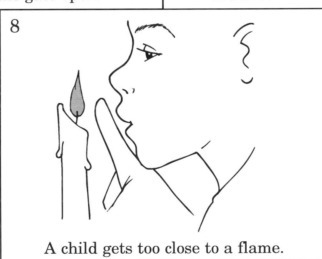

8

A child gets too close to a flame.

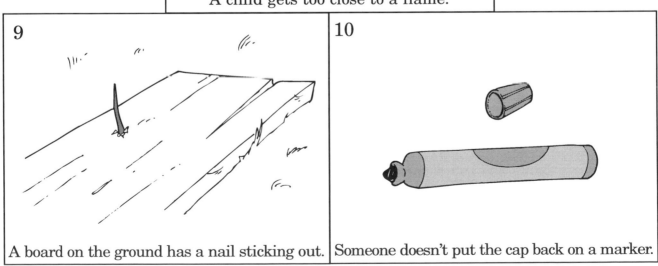

9	10
A board on the ground has a nail sticking out.	Someone doesn't put the cap back on a marker.

Answer Key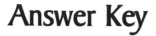

Fluency

Borderline/Mild Disfluency (pages 10–17)
Targets listed in text.

Moderate to Severe Disfluency (pages 18–23)
Targets listed in text.

Narrative/Expository — Kindergarten

Baselines 1- 4 (page 25)

> *Note:* The stories on this page and page 142 are examples of Baseline 4 stories. Baselines 1-3 would typically be in simpler form as indicated below.

Baseline 1: The student puts the pictures in the order indicated in the story below and/or on page 142.

Baseline 2: The student tells a simpler version of the story below and/or on page 142, but includes the sequence words.

Baseline 3: The student talks about the problem and solution in a simpler version of the story below and/or on page 142.

Baseline 4: The student tells a story comparable to the story below and/or on page 142.

Page 125
First the man pours water in a glass. He is thirsty. Next he accidentally knocks the glass with his elbow. The glass breaks into lots of pieces when it hits the floor. It makes a loud noise. The man feels silly because he wasn't careful. Then he cleans up the glass with a dustpan.

Page 126
First a boy is walking along on the sidewalk. He is smiling. He doesn't see the gum on the sidewalk. Next he steps on the gum and it gets stuck to his shoe. After that he leans on the fence and looks at his shoe. Last he takes off his shoe and uses a stick to scrape off the gum.

Page 127
First a girl tries to reach a book on the top shelf. She is not tall enough. Next she gets a stepstool and moves it in front of the shelf. After that she climbs on the stepstool and reaches the book. She is glad she has her book. Now she can read.

Page 128
First a girl puts the pieces of a puzzle together. The puzzle is of a puppy. She is almost finished. Next she sees that she is missing a piece. After that she looks under the table and finds the last piece. Then she puts it in the puzzle.

Page 129
First a boy is writing with a pencil. Next his pencil breaks. After that he goes to the pencil sharpener and sharpens the pencil. Then he goes back to his seat and writes again.

Page 130
First a girl rides her bike on a dirt path. Then her bike tire hits a rock and she falls off of her bike. She looks at her knee and it is cut. She feels sad because it hurts. After she gets home, she tells her mom about her hurt knee. Last her mom puts a bandage on her knee. The girl feels much better.

Page 131
First a little puppy crosses the street. Then a man looks at the puppy's collar to see where the puppy lives. After that the man finds the address and knocks on the door. Next a woman opens the door. She is happy to see her puppy. The puppy is glad to see her too.

Page 132

First a boy is walking toward a door. Next he pushes on the door, but it is too heavy. He can't open it. After that an older boy sees him and helps him push on the door. Last the door opens and they both walk outside.

Page 133

First a girl is wearing a hat with a flower on it. Then the wind blows the hat off her head. The hat lands in a tree. The girl is not tall enough to get her hat. Next she asks her dad to get her hat. He is tall so he reaches up and gets the hat out of the tree. Last he gives her hat back. The girl is happy. She says, "Thank you."

Page 134

First a girl is dribbling a basketball in her driveway. There are some tall bushes along her driveway and behind the basketball hoop. She shoots the basketball at the hoop, but the ball doesn't come back down. It is stuck. Then she goes to the garage and gets a broom. After that she stands on her tiptoes to hit the ball with the broom. Last the ball falls. She is glad that she can play basketball again.

Narrative/Expository — 1st and 2nd Grade

Baselines 1-5 (pages 26–30)

A. 1. Ben got a book from his mom.
    2. characters: Ben, his mom, his sister
        setting: home
        problem: Ben can't find his new book.
        attempt: searched all over the house
        solution: found book in sister's room
    3.-4. Accept any reasonable responses.
    5. Answers will vary.
B. 1. climbing something like a tree, ladder, or fence
    2. characters: Brad, stepdad Tim, coach, doctor
        setting: home, doctor's office, baseball field
        problem: broken ankle, baseball tryouts
        attempt: go to tryouts anyway
        solution: coach let Brad join the team without trying out
    3.-4. Accept any reasonable responses.
    5. Answers will vary.
C. 1. some kind of bird
    2. characters: Yoshi, his bird, his mom
        setting: Yoshi's home
        initiating event: bird flew into plate and broke it
        solution: bird stays in cage
    3.-4. Accept any reasonable responses.
    5. Answers will vary.
D. 1. red
    2. characters: Ashley, Jeff
        setting: outside their house, hardware store
        initiating event: painted tree house, but paint washed off with rain
        solution: painted again with outdoor paint
    3.-4. Accept any reasonable responses.
    5. Answers will vary.
E. 1. quarter got lost
    2. character: Alex
        setting: outside, school, store
        initiating event: dropped quarter he needed for soda
        solution: found empty soda cans, turned in for money, and bought soda
    3.-4. Accept any reasonable responses.
    5. Answers will vary.

F. 1. Shelly and Rosa got caught in the rain.
    2. characters: Shelly, Rosa
        setting: way home from school, their houses
        initiating event: got rained on, lost key while running
        solution: went to Rosa's house, called Shelly's mom, got warm in front of the heater
    3.-4. Accept any reasonable responses.
    5. Answers will vary.
G. 1. in an airplane
    2. characters: Anna, flight attendant
        setting: airplane
        initiating event: Anna saw her house, but flight attendant didn't recognize name of street
        solution: showed attendant street on map
    3.-4. Accept any reasonable responses.
    5. Answers will vary.
H. 1. a cow
    2. characters: Sarah, cow, snake
        setting: field
        initiating event: cow saw snake
        solution: Sarah screamed and the snake slithered away.
    3.-4. Accept any reasonable responses.
    5. Answers will vary.
I. 1. to replace the window they broke while playing softball
    2. characters: Rachel, Melanie, Rachel's dad
        setting: house, store
        initiating event: broke window playing softball
        solution: sold toys to earn money to replace window
    3.-4. Accept any reasonable responses.
    5. Answers will vary.
J. 1. Mr. Jacoby adopted it.
    2. characters: Mr. Jacoby, cat, children
        setting: neighborhood
        initiating event: Mr. Jacoby was lonely.
        solution: adopted a cat that made him feel happy

Narrative/Expository — 3rd and 4th Grade

Baseline 1 (page 31)
Targets listed in text.

Baseline 2 (page 31)
Answers will vary.

Baseline 3 (pages 31–33)
  1. yellow and pink
      the sunset
      cotton candy
      evening

  2. squeaking
      one hand on the cart and one hand holding the list
      gray
      hard, because one wheel was off balance

  3. on its side
      scraps of food
      large
      unsure because he kept looking around

4. dark gray or black
   tall corn blowing in the wind, clouds moving across the sky, flashes of lightning
   thunder and heavy rain
   in the country because there are cornfields

5. ten
   a birthday
   a girl
   a child because there are only 10 candles

6. a quilt
   Her hands hurt.
   She might not be able to finish the quilt by winter.
   October or November

7. excited
   runners running
   red
   running shorts, tank tops, socks, and shoes

8. brown and white
   jumping puppy
   restless
   wants to play

9. sizzling
   black
   yellow, golden brown
   square

10. daytime, noon
    white, green
    calm
    It snowed.

Baseline 4 (page 34)
1. the Chinese
2. songs
3. Melinda
4. hundreds of people
5. the passenger's
6. Zac's book on table
7. the woman who called
8. the flower
9. the lion and tiger
10. the burglar

Baseline 5 (pages 34–35)
Answers listed in text.

Narrative/Expository — 5th and 6th Grade

Baselines 1-4 (pages 36–37)
Answers will vary.

Narrative/Expository — 7th – 12th Grade

Baselines 1-2 (pages 38–39)
Answers will vary.

Baselines 3-4 (pages 39–41)
Answers listed in text.

Oral-Motor/Articulation

Oral-Motor Skills

Baselines 1-5 (page 43)
Targets described in text.

Articulation Skills

Baselines 1-7 (page 44)
Targets described in text.

Student/Parent/Teacher Involvement

Baselines 1-4 (page 45)
Targets described in text.

Phonological Awareness — K – 2nd Grade

Baseline 1 (page 47)
Answers will vary.

Baselines 2-3A (pages 47–48)
Answers listed in text.

Baseline 3B (page 49)
1. end with /p/
2. begin with /m/
3. end with /ee/
4. end with /l/
5. begin with /k/
6. begin with /s/
7. begin with /f/
8. begin with /d/
9. begin with /w/
10. end with /n/

Baselines 4–6 (pages 49–50)
Answers listed in text.

Pragmatics — K – 6th Grade

Baseline 1 (pages 52–54)
Answers will vary.

Baseline 2 (page 55)
Targets listed in text.

Pragmatics — 7th – 12th Grade

Baselines 1–2 (pages 56–57)
Answers will vary.

Semantics — Kindergarten

Baseline 1 (page 59)
1. They are all fruits except the carrots. Carrots are vegetables.
2. They are all numbers except the *B*. A *B* is a letter.
3. They are all farm animals except the zebra. A zebra is a zoo or jungle animal.
4. They are all things to ride in except the wheel. A wheel is only part of something to ride in.
5. They are all things to read except the desk. A desk is where you sit to write or read.
6. They are all things a baby would use except the glass. A glass is something bigger children and adults drink from.
7. They are all things that give light except the phone. You talk on a phone.
8. They are all things to write with except the paints. You use paints to color a picture.
9. They are all things that fly except the tree. A tree grows in the ground.
10. They are all things to eat with except the saw. You cut with a saw.

Baseline 2 (page 59)
Answers listed in text.

Baseline 3 (page 59)
1. The ice cream fell off the cone because the girl accidentally turned it sideways.
2. The tire is flat because when someone was riding the bike he ran over a nail and the tire popped.
3. The window is broken because some kids were playing baseball in the backyard. One of them hit the ball through the window and it landed on the floor.
4. The toast is burned because someone left it in too long and it got too hot.
5. No one remembered to water the flower in the pot so it got really dry.
6. No one can swing on the swing because the chain broke. Maybe someone who was too heavy sat in it and broke it.
7. The water is leaking out of the bucket because there is a crack in it.
8. The puppy got stuck in the opening because he is too big.
9. Nobody cleared the table because the family had to leave in a hurry.
10. No one can rake the leaves because the rake is broken.

Baseline 4 (page 59)
1. She might get sick.
2. He might get hurt.
3. The sink will overflow and water will spill onto the floor.
4. The TV won't work.
5. The Popsicle will melt/get sticky.
6. The dog could get out/get lost.
7. The balloon will pop.
8. The boy might burn himself.
9. Someone could step on it and get hurt.
10. The marker will dry out/not work.

Semantics — 1st and 2nd Grade

Baseline 1 (pages 60–62)
1. a
2. b
3. c
4. b
5. c
6. c

7. a
8. c
9. a
10. b

Baseline 2 (pages 62–63)
Answers will vary.

Baselines 3-4 (page 63)
Answers listed in text.

Baseline 5 (page 64)
1. Sarah felt embarrassed that she had to go around with a stain on her sweater.
2. Michael gets up early on his birthday so he can have a long time to celebrate.
3. We had bumps because we got bit by the mosquitoes.
4. The bear went to the stream because he knew there were fish there to eat.
5. She put cotton in her ears so the talking wouldn't bother her.
6. The eggs broke because they hit the ground when the wind knocked them out of the tree.
7. Tannen fell down because his shoelace was too long/untied and he tripped on it.
8. Amy was afraid because she couldn't see anything in the dark and felt like something bad could happen.
9. Patrice climbed into her grandma's lap because she wanted to listen to a story.
10. His pants were green because the wet paint got on them when he sat down.

Baseline 6 (pages 64–65)
1. fish
2. look
3. how far
4. shy
5. the bottom
6. pieces
7. jobs
8. tired
9. strange
10. well-known

Baseline 7 (pages 66–68)
Answers will vary for Quantity, Spatial, Ordinal, and Operations sections. Answers listed in text for Temporal section.

Semantics — 3rd and 4th Grade

Baselines 1-6 (pages 69–74)
A. 1. the good things about new ideas that people have
   2. New ideas make life better.
   3. Accept any three or four important details from the passage.
   4. *innovation* or *innovator*. If the student responds "no," probe for understanding of *innovation* or *innovator*. If the student cannot define it or use an example from the text, the benchmark has not been met.
   5. noun
   6. a person who invents something

B. 1. the first people to live in America; Native Americans
   2. People came to America to have a better life.
   3. Accept any three or four important details from the passage.
   4. *immigrants*
   5. noun
   6. people who came from another country

C. 1. doing something better in space; hot air balloons; aircraft
   2. The *Voyager* was the first airplane to fly around the world without stopping.
   3. Accept any three or four important details from the passage.
   4. *mission*
   5. noun
   6. goal of the trip

D. 1. a family tree; old photographs; discovery of the camera
   2. The camera went through many changes.
   3. Accept any three or four important details from the passage.
   4. *negative*
   5. noun
   6. a copy of the image on film

E. 1. something interesting about the brain
   2. The brain can do amazing things.
   3. Accept any three or four important details from the passage.
   4. *incredible*
   5. adjective
   6. unbelievable; hard to imagine

F. 1. information about a certain kind of dog/terriers
   2. Terriers can be helpful dogs.
   3. Accept any three or four important details from the passage.
   4. *game*
   5. noun
   6. animals hunted/killed for food

G. 1. somewhere people like to visit in Delaware
   2. A lot of people live around Wilmington.
   3. Accept any three or four important details from the passage.
   4. *metropolitan*
   5. adjective
   6. consisting of a big city and its suburbs

H. 1. someone who wrote books a lot of people like to read
   2. Charles Dickens wrote many books that a lot of people like.
   3. Accept any three or four important details from the passage.
   4. *novelist*
   5. noun
   6. an author

I. 1. how dolphins talk
   2. Dolphins have their own way of talking to each other.
   3. Accept any three or four important details from the passage.
   4. *system*
   5. noun
   6. way of doing something

J. 1. what farm animals eat
   2. Hay is used to feed farm animals.
   3. Accept any three or four important details from the passage.
   4. *bales*
   5. verb
   6. to put the hay into bundles

Semantics — 5th and 6th Grade

Baseline 1 (page 75)
1. very large; too big for someone to eat by himself
2. home; out of school; to sports practice
3. brown
4. in an airplane
5. baseball field
6. bank teller
7. midnight
8. to a fire; to an emergency
9. big and strong
10. She was really hungry.

Baselines 2-7 (pages 76–81)
A. 2. bad or negative things that could happen if trees are cut down
   3. Cutting down forests causes serious damage.
   4. Accept any four important details from the passage.
   5. *deforestation*
   6. noun
   7. trees cut/forests cleared

B. 2. the weather patterns of China like temperature, etc.
   3. China has many different climates.
   4. Accept any four important details from the passage.
   5. *diverse*
   6. adjective
   7. different

C. 2. when the yo-yo was first invented/made
   3. The yo-yo was used as a tool when it was first created.
   4. Accept any four important details from the passage.
   5. *retrieve*
   6. verb
   7. get it back

D. 2. facts about history
   3. Archeologists use artifacts to learn about the past.
   4. Accept any four important details from the passage.
   5. *artifacts*
   6. noun
   7. objects from long ago used to find out about the past

E. 2. how to know if something is true/real
   3. There are differences between fact and reasoned judgment.
   4. Accept any four important details from the passage.
   5. *validated*
   6. verb
   7. to prove something

F. 2. information about whales (e.g., their size or where they live)
   3. The blue whale is the largest living creature.
   4. Accept any four important details from the passage.
   5. *immense*
   6. adjective
   7. huge, enormous

G. 2. ways the snow can be dangerous (e.g., snowstorms or avalanches)
    3. An avalanche can be dangerous to anything in its path.
    4. Accept any four important details from the passage.
    5. *tremendous*
    6. adjective
    7. a lot; a great amount of

H. 2. something we don't think of as friendly; a friend we didn't know about
    3. Bats are creatures that are helpful to humans.
    4. Accept any four important details from the passage.
    5. *reputation*
    6. noun
    7. known for

I. 2. something to do that can cool you off; something fun to do in the summer
    3. Tubing is popular in the summer.
    4. Accept any four important details from the passage.
    5. *suitable*
    6. adjective
    7. appropriate; it "works"; it's okay

J. 2. information about trails in the hills/dirt roads; how to bike off the road, etc.
    3. BMX biking is a fun sport.
    4. Accept any four important details from the passage.
    5. *rugged*
    6. adjective
    7. not smooth; bumpy; uneven

Baseline 8 (pages 81–82)
Answers listed in text.

Semantics — 7th – 12th Grade

Baselines 1-3 (pages 83–86)
A. 1. Ulama was an Aztec ball game.
    2. Accept any four important details from the passage.
    3. push, move

B. 1. "Blistering" was used in early medicine.
    2. Accept any four important details from the passage.
    3. way of doing something

C. 1. House designs copied Gothic buildings during the Victorian era.
    2. Accept any four important details from the passage.
    3. ugly

D. 1. Tests on treadmills are used to measure fitness.
    2. Accept any four important details from the passage.
    3. difficult

E. 1. Before mattresses, people slept on straw.
    2. Accept any four important details from the passage.
    3. something that supports

F. 1. Dogs display their feelings through their body language.
    2. Accept any four important details from the passage.
    3. emotions; how someone (or a dog) feels; attitude

G. 1. Expansion happens when molecules are heated.
    2. Accept any four important details from the passage.
    3. loosely

H. 1. Although we're trying to reduce pollution, it is still a major problem.
    2. Accept any four important details from the passage.
    3. swallowed, taken into the body

I. 1. Writing from long ago is hard to read.
    2. Accept any four important details from the passage.
    3. type of paper

J. 1. The Sahara is the world's largest desert.
    2. Accept any four important details from the passage.
    3. able to grow something; give life

Baseline 4 (pages 86–89)
Answers listed in text.

Baseline 5 (pages 89–93)

1.

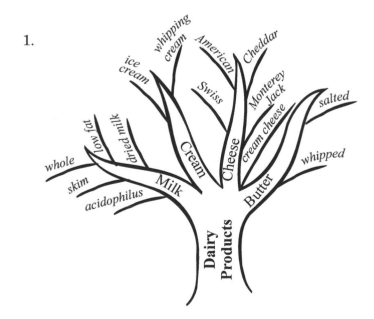

2.

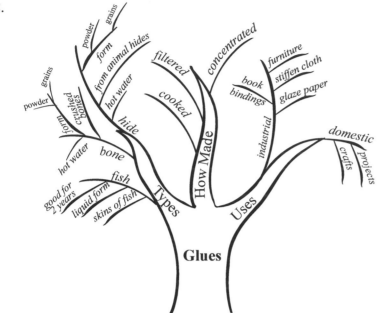

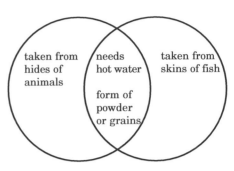

hide glue   bone glue

3.

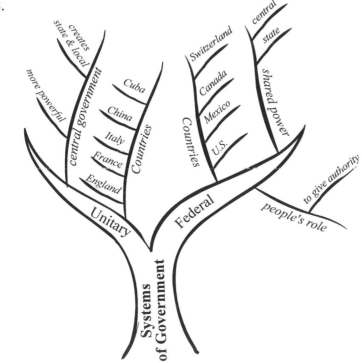

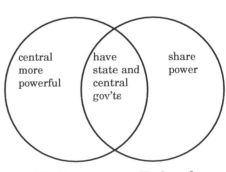

Unitary   Federal

4.

5.

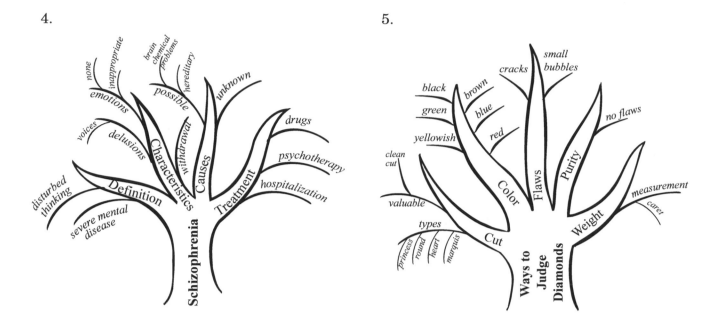

6.

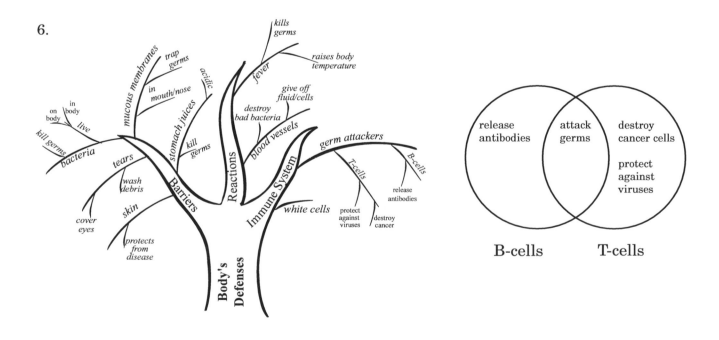

7.

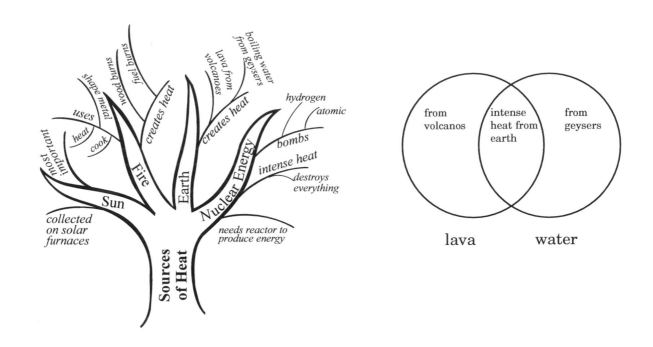

Sources of Heat

Fire — wood burns, fuel burns, creates heat
- uses, important, heat, cook, shape metal
Sun — important, collected on solar furnaces
Earth — creates heat, lava from volcanoes, boiling water from geysers
Nuclear Energy — hydrogen, atomic, bombs, intense heat, destroys everything, needs reactor to produce energy

Venn diagram:
- lava: from volcanos
- intense heat from earth
- water: from geysers

8.

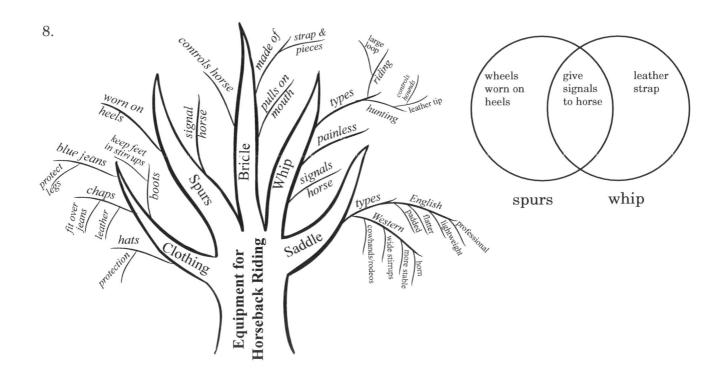

Equipment for Horseback Riding

Clothing — worn on heels, blue jeans, protect legs, chaps, fit over jeans, leather, hats, protection
Spurs — keep feet in stirrups, boots, signal horse
Bricle — controls horse, made of, strap & pieces, pulls on mouth
Whip — types, large loop, riding, controls hounds, leather tip, hunting, painless, signals horse
Saddle — types, English, professional, flatter, lightweight, padded, Western, cowhands/rodeos, wide stirrups, more stable, horn

Venn diagram:
- spurs: wheels worn on heels
- give signals to horse
- whip: leather strap

9.

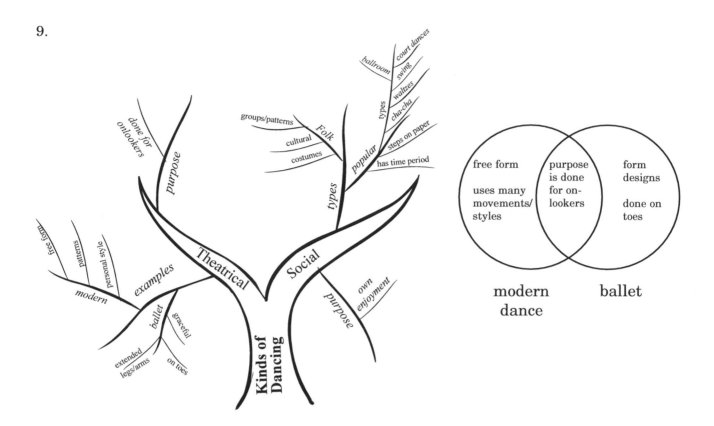

10.

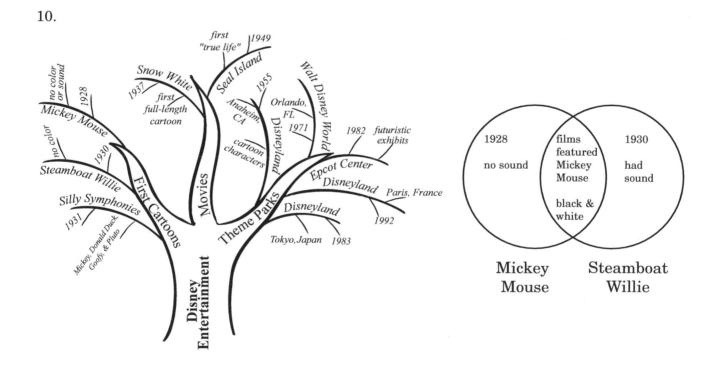

Baseline 6 (pages 93–94)
1. bleak, dreary, dark, overcast
2. weak, sickly, fragile, feeble
3. strong, sturdy, tight
4. excuse, argument, cause
5. excited, anxious, tense
6. encouraged, backed, defended
7. still, quiet, smooth
8. tied, matched, the same
9. decide, rule, determine
10. prank, mischief, trick

Syntax — Kindergarten

Baselines 1-5 (pages 96–98)
Answers listed in text.

Syntax — 1st Grade

Baselines 1-2 (page 99)
Answers listed in text.

Syntax — 2nd Grade

Baselines 1-3 (page 100)
Answers listed in text.

Syntax — 3rd and 4th Grade

Baseline 1 (page 101)
Answers listed in text.

Baseline 2 (pages 101–102)
1. same
2. different
3. different
4. same
5. same
6. different
7. same
8. different
9. same
10. different

Baseline 3 (page 102)
1. The book bag was carried by the man.
2. The computer keyboard was hit by her.
3. The flowers in the yard were picked by Andrea.
4. The cat was fed by Lauri.
5. Her daughter was taken to the zoo by Maureen.
6. The gas bill was paid by Joe.
7. The anchor was pulled out of the water by Karen.
8. The letter was mailed by Jackie.
9. The lawn was mowed yesterday by André.
10. The new car was driven by Tony.

Baselines 4-5 (pages 102–103)
Answers will vary.

Baseline 6 (page 103)
Possible answers:
1. Mena *softly* read the story.
2. Jeremy jumped *proudly* over the hurdle.
3. The book fell *noisily* to the ground.
4. The horse bucked *wildly*.
5. Fish swim *energetically* upstream.
6. The boy *carefully* cut the ribbon.
7. She watched *patiently* as the fish neared her hook.
8. The teacher spoke *harshly* to the rowdy students.
9. He *quickly* untied the rope.
10. Pete sang *loudly* over the music.

Baseline 7 (page 104)
1. imperative because someone is being told to do something
2. exclamatory because it shows strong feeling about the size of the crown
3. interrogative because someone is asking a question
4. declarative because someone is making a statement
5. exclamatory because it shows strong feeling
6. imperative because someone is being told not to do something
7. exclamatory because it shows strong feeling
8. imperative because someone is being told not to forget
9. interrogative because someone is asking a question
10. declarative because someone made a statement

Baseline 8 (pages 104–106)
Possible answers are listed in the text.

Syntax — 5th and 6th Grade

Baseline 1 (page 107)
1. An opossum was found.
   Its mother was killed by a car.
   It is 4 weeks old.
   It has to be fed with a tiny bottle.
   It is at the California Wildlife Center.

2. Washington High School has a $2 million air-conditioning system.
   There is some kind of problem with the air-conditioning system.
   The parents are complaining about it.
   The school will replace most of the system.

3. Most states have inspections of their theme parks.
   In most states, theme parks have to show records of accidents.
   Twelve states don't have rules about this.
   California is one of these states.

4. The Lexington Library will make an announcement.
   The announcement will be today.
   It has acquired writings.
   It has all the writings.
   The writings are from Felix Hebert.
   Felix Hebert was born in Britain.

5. Video game sales are growing fast.
   People usually spend more money on movies than video games.
   People will probably spend more on video games than movies this year.
   This is the first time that has ever happened.

6. There was a fire in November.
   It destroyed one-fourth of the Wharf.
   The Wharf was the city's biggest attraction.
   It has been hard to find the cause of the fire.
   Rebuilding the Wharf hasn't been very difficult.

7. There was a wreck.
   There were passengers hurt.
   Some injuries were serious; some were minor.
   Most of the people hurt were women.
   The women were in their 70s and 80s.

8. There was a case.
   The case involved a robbery.
   The case has gone to a grand jury.
   The grand jury is made up of people from San Antonio.
   The Dallas Daily News reported the details.

9. Spears College will play a baseball game.
   The game will be a playoff.
   The game will be the first one in the playoffs.
   There will be six teams in the playoffs.
   The game is against Charter University.
   The game will be played in Idaho.

10. There was an accident.
    It was a hit-and-run.
    The driver hit a parked car.
    Deputies are investigating the accident.
    The deputies are from the Sheriff's Office.

Baseline 2 (pages 108–109)
Accept any reasonable responses.

Baseline 3 (page 109)
Answers will vary.

Syntax — 7th – 12th Grade

Baseline 1 (pages 110–113)
Temporal
1. Answer listed in text.
2. *Before* the War of 1887, the country was under communist rule.
3. *While* the citizens marched outside the building, the mayor met with city officials.
4. *After* Catherine the Great came to power, Russia had great success.
5. He spent five years in Vermont as a child, *then* he moved to New Hampshire in his teenage years.

Causal
1. Answer listed in text.
2. The air had a strange smell *so* the students reported it to their teacher.
3. *Because* some people who run like to watch TV while they exercise, fitness clubs have placed TV sets above the treadmill equipment.
4. He borrowed from a friend *because* he didn't have enough money with him to pay for lunch.
5. The book had a stain on the cover *so* she asked the clerk to give her a discount on the price.

Conditional
1. Answer listed in text.
2. Dance schools will have to increase the number of instructors *if* ballet becomes popular with more teenagers.
3. *If* gas continues to get more expensive, more people may carpool.
4. The measure would have passed *if* more Americans knew about the issue.
5. *If* there is a positive review of the film, it will be shown as part of a class assignment.

Notice-Perception
1. Answer listed in text.
2. 1948, *when* Israel became a nation, remains an important date in Israel's history.
3. New Zealand, *where* outdoor activities are popular, held the largest teddy bear picnic in 1994.
4. Vegetation is plentiful in the coastal region *where* the soil is fertile.
5. The famous baseball player, *who* just beat the world's record for the fastest pitch, gave a press conference.

Specification
1. Answer listed in text.
2. The popular television show *that* starred Martha Long lasted until 1978.
3. The MVP award, *which* is the most popular, was given to Reggie Simmons.
4. The dance called the waltz, *which* was first danced in England, was outlawed in some places at first.
5. The Central Union Pacific Railroad, *which* was finished in 1869, was the first to extend from coast to coast.

Adversative
1. Answer listed in text.
2. His father took him to see the movie last year, *but* he forgot the main characters.
3. *Even though* the concert was for a good cause, it was still expensive.
4. The store had a clearance sale on jackets, *but* it only lasted three hours.
5. *Although* the new mayor seemed to be popular, she only won the election by 50 votes.

Baseline 2 (pages 113–114)
Answers will vary.

Baseline 3 (page 114)
Answers listed in text.

Voice — Education

Baselines 1-8 (pages 116 –118)
Targets listed in text.

Voice — Treatment

Baselines 1-2 (page 119)
Targets listed in text.

Baseline 3 (pages 119–120)
Accept reasonable productions.

Word-Finding

Baselines 1-3 (pages 122–124)
Answers listed in text.

Baseline 4 (page 124)
Accept any reasonable answers.

Baseline 5 (page 124)
Answers listed in text.

References

Armento, B. J., Klor de Alva, J. J., Nash, G. B., Salter, C. L., Wilson, L. E., and Wixson, K. K. *A Message of Ancient Days*. Boston, MA: Houghton Mifflin Company, 1994.

Ad Hoc Committee on the Roles and Responsibilities of the School-Based Speech-Language Pathologist. "Guidelines for the Roles and Responsibilities of the School-Based Speech-Language Pathologist." *ASHA Handbook*, Approved March 1999.

American-Speech-Language-Hearing Association Committee on Policy & Legislation. "Case Position on Benchmarks." *ASHA Leader*, Oct. 6, 1998.

Bankson, N. and Bernthal, J. *Articulation and Phonological Disorders*. Englewood Cliffs, NJ: Prentice Hall, 1988.

Bell, N. *Visualizing and Verbalizing for Language Comprehension and Thinking*. Paso Robles, CA: Academy of Reading Publications, 1991.

Benson, B. E. and Rees, P. W. "Delaware." In *World Book Encyclopedia*. Chicago, IL: World Book, Inc., 1998.

Berman, S. S. *Phonology for Groups: Thematic Activities for Everyday Settings*. San Antonio: Communication Skill Builders, a division of The Psychological Corporation, 1996.

Bernger, P. A. "Schizophrenia." In *World Book Encyclopedia*. Chicago, IL: World Book, Inc., 1998.

Boning, R. *Specific Skills Series*. New York: Barnell Loft, Ltd., 1977.

Boshart, C. A. *Essential Oral-Motor Techniques*. Temecula, CA: Speech Dynamics, 1997.

California State Board of Education. *California Language Arts Content Standards*. "Reading, writing, written and oral English language conventions, and listening and speaking for grades K-12." Sacramento, CA: 1988.

Collins, K. K. "Charles Dickens." In *World Book Encyclopedia*. Chicago, IL: World Book, Inc., 1998.

Fenner, C. "The Skates of Uncle Richard." In *Rolling Waves*. McGraw-Hill Reading Series. Oklahoma City, OK: McGraw-Hill, Inc., 1989.

Ferguson, M., Hoskins, B., and Montgomery, J. "IDEA '97: Reframing Your Role and Focusing on the Curriculum." Workshop presented at the California Speech-Language-Hearing Association Conference, Sacramento, CA: April 1999.

Fisher, D. "Dolphins." In *World Book Encyclopedia*. Chicago, IL: World Book, Inc., 1998.

Fosnot, S. M. *Fluency Development in Young Stutterers: Differential Diagnosis and Treatment*. The Riverside Publishing Company, Itasca, IL: 1992.

Fox, M. W. "Dogs." In *World Book Encyclopedia*. Chicago, IL: World Book, Inc., 1998.

Georgia's Quality Core Curriculum. 11 November, 1999 <http://admin.doe.K12.ga.US/gadoe/sla/qcccopy.nsf>

Givón, T. *English Grammar: A Function-Based Introduction*. Philadelphia, PA: John Benjamins, 1993.

Hill, D., Gregory, H., Bernstein-Ratner, N., Yaruss, J. S., Chmela, K., Campbell, J. H., and Gregory, C. "Stuttering Therapy: A Workshop for Specialists." Workshop presented in Chicago, IL and sponsored by Northwestern University and The Stuttering Foundation of America, July 14-25, 1997.

Hutjens, M. F. "Dairy." In *World Book Encyclopedia*. Chicago, IL: World Book, Inc., 1998.

Katz, S. L. and English, P. C. "Disease." In *World Book Encyclopedia*. Chicago, IL: World Book, Inc., 1998.

Keets, E. J. "Wake the Sun." In *Peter's Chair*. McGraw-Hill Reading Series. Oklahoma City, OK: McGraw-Hill, Inc., 1989.

Lawson, R. "Ben and Me." In *Dreams Go Far*. McGraw-Hill Reading Series. Oklahoma City, OK: McGraw-Hill, Inc., 1989.

Maloy, J. "The Winter Sleep." In *Upon a Shore*. McGraw-Hill Reading Series. Oklahoma City, OK: McGraw-Hill, Inc., 1989.

Nelson, N. W. *Childhood Language Disorders in Context: Infancy Through Adolescence*. New York: Macmillan Co., 1993.

Nelson, R. P. "Walt Disney." In *World Book Encyclopedia*. Chicago, IL: World Book, Inc., 1998.

Odom, S. O. "Dance." In *World Book Encyclopedia*. Chicago, IL: World Book, Inc., 1998.

Paul, R. *Language Disorders from Infancy Through Adolescence: Assessment and Intervention*. New York: Mosby, 1995.

Plass, B. *SPARC R*. East Moline, IL: LinguiSystems, Inc., 1994.

Plass, B. *SPARC S*. East Moline, IL: LinguiSystems, Inc., 1994.

Plass, B. *SPARC L*. East Moline, IL: LinguiSystems, Inc., 1994.

Pough, F. H. "Diamonds." In *World Book Encyclopedia*. Chicago, IL: World Book, Inc., 1998.

Price, S. D. and Landsman, B. "Horse." In *World Book Encyclopedia*. Chicago, IL: World Book, Inc., 1998.

Ramig, P., Guitar, B., Healey, C., Murphy, B., Chmela, K., and Reardon, N. "Stuttering Therapy: Practical Ideas for the School Clinician." Workshop presented in Newport Beach, CA and sponsored by The Stuttering Foundation of America, Chapman University, and California Speech-Language-Hearing Association, June 5-6, 1998.

Rieck, J. N. "Glue." In *World Book Encyclopedia*. Chicago, IL: World Book, Inc., 1998.

Saugus Union School District. *English Language Arts Content Standards: Kindergarten through Sixth Grade*. Saugus, CA: Adopted 1998.

Saugus Union School District. *Mathematics Content Standards: Kindergarten through Sixth Grade*. Saugus, CA: Adopted 1998.

Schenone, L. and Garbarini, P. "Just the Thing." In *City Magic*. McGraw-Hill Reading Series. Oklahoma City, OK: McGraw-Hill, Inc., 1989.

Scott, C. "Fill the Sky." In *The Mystery of Corbin Lodge*. McGraw-Hill Reading Series. Oklahoma City, OK: McGraw-Hill, Inc., 1989.

Simms, S. R. *"Say and Do" Mazes for Articulation*. Greenville, SC: Super Duper School Company, 1997.

Squire, C. F. "Heat." In *World Book Encyclopedia*. Chicago, IL: World Book, Inc., 1998.

Thomsen, S. *SPARC Revised*. East Moline, IL: LinguiSystems, Inc., 1994.

Vermeer, D. V. "Sahara Desert." In *World Book Encyclopedia*. Chicago, IL: World Book, Inc., 1998.

Webber, M. T. Jr. and Webber, S. G. *Webber's Jumbo Articulation Drill Book*. Greenville, SC: Super Duper School Company, 1993.

Weidenbaum, M. L. "Government." In *World Book Encyclopedia*. Chicago, IL: World Book, Inc., 1998.

Wilson, K. D. *Voice Problems of Children: Third Edition*. Los Angeles, CA: Williams & Wilkins, 1987.